Journey to Authenticity

VOICES OF CHIEF RESIDENTS

Edited by Julie A. Jacob

Photography by Roberta E. Sonnino, MD

Preface by David C. Leach, MD

Accreditation Council for Graduate Medical Education

© 2007 Accreditation Council for Graduate Medical Education

Printed in the United States of America.
All rights reserved.

Additional copies of this book may be ordered by contacting the ACGME.

Editor: Julie A. Jacob

Design: Arc Group Ltd, Chicago

Photography: HiRES Photos
except page 64, courtesy of the U.S. Navy; page 65, Michael Frew;
pages 108–109, Terry Dagradi, MedMedia Group, Yale School of Medicine.

ISBN: 0-9794018-0-1
        978-0-9794018-0-0

ACKNOWLEDGEMENTS

The ACGME thanks the physicians who graciously shared their resident experiences for this book and Dr. Roberta Sonnino, who volunteered her time and tirelessly traveled across the country to photograph the chief residents.

CONTENTS

Preface   6

PRIMARY CARE PHYSICIANS

Jessica O'Leary Burness, MD   10

Jennifer M. Weiss, MD   16

Lanessa D. Bass, MD   22

Mari A. Ricker, MD   28

Thomas Renaud, MD   32

Brandi W. Trammell, MD   38

SURGEONS

Shahab Abdessalam, MD   46

Gil Binenbaum, MD   52

Vishal C. Gala, MD, MPH   58

Theresa L. Castro, MD   64

Bryan B. Voelzke, MD   72

Charlotte Eielson Ariyan, MD, PhD   78

Clifford M. Perez, MD   84

SPECIALISTS

Samuel K. Caughron, MD   90

Kathleen Ang-Lee, MD   96

Robert J. Gore, MD   100

Benjamin D. Smith, MD   108

Jill Weinstein, MD   114

Cynthia L. Bodkin, MD   118

Reed M. VanMatre, MD   124

PREFACE

There is no steeper learning curve in medicine than residency. The dramatic differences between interns and chief residents can only be described as a journey to authenticity, a journey in which physicians discover both clinical wisdom and themselves. It is a journey that no one can take for them or spare them; it is a journey that is surrounded by external drama, but which actually proceeds from the inside out. It is a journey that calls on the intellect but also the will and the imagination. Residents learn to discern and tell the truth but also to make good clinical judgments in ways that are sometimes creative and even beautiful. It is the reason they went into medicine.

This small volume offers a biopsy of the experience; it captures a few stories about some remarkable people. We can see the process through their eyes and get a glimpse of what is really going on. Educators would tell us that what is going on is a shift from rule-based behavior to context-based behavior. Junior physicians learn the rules of medicine; in residency one applies those rules to different and increasingly complex cases and learns that the particulars of the patient are as important as, and frequently more important than, the rules. Residency calls on art as well as science. The resident not only needs to know about pneumonia, but also when Mary Smith gets pneumonia they need to know about Mary Smith. The rules about pneumonia are generalizable; Mary Smith is unique. Context is important.

Most physicians can describe the first patient they saw as residents and they can describe them in great detail, even though it may have been thirty years ago. The experience is seared into doctors' brains in a very special way. While the science of medicine changes (it is in the nature of science to ever more closely approximate the truth but never actually get there), it is the stories that are remembered. It is the stories that inform the good clinician about next steps. Yet it is common to get lost in the patients' stories – they do not proceed in a logical linear fashion, rather they move in circles and circles within circles. It is easy to get lost – learning to get lost in order to find the real truth is one of the lessons of residency.

Paying attention to patients' stories enables residents to discover their own stories. Their stories are frequently about their competence, their character and their communities. Competence is a habit. It involves more than knowledge and skill; it involves how you think as well as what you think. Competence requires values as well as rules, fidelity as well as effectiveness. Competence is the demonstrated habit of reflective practice. Chief residents are competent. In becoming competent they develop and discover their characters. Their characters, in turn, both contribute to and are shaped by the character of the community in which they are formed; hence, the ACGME's interest in residency programs.

Residents learn that medicine is a cooperative and not a productive art. They don't provide a pound of healing but rather reduce barriers to healing. They cooperate with the body's natural tendency to heal. The outcome isn't totally dependent on them. The quality of patient care depends on the quality of the relationships, relationships with patients and with colleagues and also the profession's relationship with society as a whole. Patient care is not just about naming the disease; it is about relieving the burden of illness. Sympathy is not enough. Empathy and compassion are needed. Sympathy says: "I'm sorry you feel bad." Suffering humans need more than that; they need to have their subjective feelings recognized, validated and honored. Patients benefit from the resident's objectivity, but they also benefit from their companionship in their subjectivity. Naming the disease is not the same as addressing the hurt. That is another learning chief residents have acquired.

The dictionary defines authenticity as: "… conforming to fact or reality; trustworthy, not imaginary, not false, not an imitation … bona fide." Chief residents are authentic physicians. Enjoy their stories.

David C. Leach, MD
Executive Director, ACGME

10   16   22   28

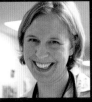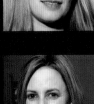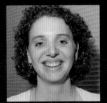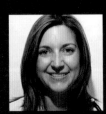

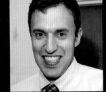

32   38

PRIMARY CARE PHYSICIANS

"It is a constant growth cycle where maybe about six or seven months into your position you start to feel a bit comfortable, but then you get new responsibilities a few months later and you feel like the new kid on the block again."

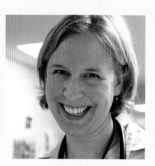

The combination of science and art is what attracted Jessica O'Leary Burness, MD, to medicine. When it was time for her to choose her specialty, it was the broad community context in which family physicians practice that made her decide to specialize in family medicine.

Although her medical career is just starting, Dr. O'Leary Burness has already demonstrated her dedication to helping people who are underserved in health care. While a medical student at Brown University School of Medicine, she helped create a free student-run community health clinic and volunteered at hospitals in Costa Rica and Kenya. Following the end of her chief residency in 2005, Dr. O'Leary Burness split her year between locums with the Multnomah County Health Department in Portland, inpatient and emergency room practice in Kotzebue, Alaska, and inpatient pediatrics through the Yale/Johnson and Johnson International Scholars Program in Livingstone, Zambia.

She recently began practicing at the Native American Rehabilitation Center Clinic in Portland where she practices outpatient adult, pediatric, and geriatric medicine and provides prenatal care.

In her free time, Dr. O'Leary Burness likes to read, write, cook, hike and bicycle.

Why did you decide to become a physician?

When I was younger, I wanted to be a teacher, an author, a museum curator or a veterinarian for endangered species. When I was 17, very suddenly during a conversation with a friend — I am not even sure what we were talking about, it was pretty random — it just hit me that medicine made sense. It is the perfect melding of literary and humanistic issues and skills with science. It is one of the few fields where there is this great integration of the sciences and humanities. That was the biggest appeal for me. It is not only a scientific field but also a melding of science and the humanities.

"You are an educator, politician,

I majored in biology at Brown University. I was also part of a liberal medical education program, which partially integrated the undergraduate and medical school years but did not accelerate the course of study. The idea was to emphasize the humanistic core of medicine.

JESSICA O'LEARY BURNESS, MD

Chief Resident, Family Medicine

Oregon Health and Sciences University

Portland, Oregon

diplomat and facilitator."

What attracted you to family medicine?

It is the only field that is rooted in the concept of treating individuals in the context of their families, communities and themselves, as opposed to focusing on any one organ or just kids or just women. It is about viewing patients as people interacting within the context of their families and communities. I liked the breadth and holistic part of it. I chose Oregon because, first, I wanted to be on the West Coast, closer to my family; second was the reputation of the family medicine program; and third, there was the program director, Dr. Eric Walsh.

What were you feeling when you started your residency?

Terror. Excitement. Hope that I would find mentors who would be inspirations. The biggest thing was that terror, that fear of not being able to be effective in the decisions. The simplest way to say it would be a fear of being a bad doctor, of making mistakes that would hurt people, of being ineffective. The fear waned — partially! — in the course of the residency.

"GENUINE CARE AND CONCERN AND TRYING YOUR BEST TO HELP IS WHAT IS TRULY IMPORTANT TO PATIENTS."

What moments from your first year stand out?

There was a very early-on case, about two months into my intern year. I had seen an elderly woman in clinic, and she had complained about a headache. I had not included temporal arteritis in my differential diagnosis. I treated her for a more traditional headache, and she ended up having a stroke as a direct result a month later. Fortunately, she recovered fully. I was completely guilt-ridden that I had missed this diagnosis. Had I not missed that diagnosis and treated her appropriately, she might not have had the event. I was just completely mortified by the whole situation. She came back to me after the diagnosis, and I told her that the headache was probably a warning sign that I should have treated her differently. I expected her to be very upset with me and, in fact, she really was not. She had no blame. She did not expect me to have made that leap, and, in fact, was very pleased that I would continue to be there for her and that I had been kind and caring and had visited her in the hospital. Medically, I had learned a lesson, and I did not want to have further missed diagnoses. I wanted to provide better technical medical care, but it was really revealing about what is truly important to patients: genuine care and concern and trying your best to help them. I learned that, while avoidance of mistakes and lifelong medical learning is critical, that mistakes in and of themselves are human and that does not make you a bad doctor, so long as you can learn from the mistakes and be honest with your patient. It was very much an eye-opening experience.

When did you start thinking of yourself as a doctor?

It happened before my residency. I spent two-and-a-half months in medical school doing inpatient medicine in Kenya, and for the most part we did not have much supervision. I was not totally on my own, but I was much more unsupervised than I had been in the United States. When I went to my residency, I felt much more confident than I would have otherwise.

What made you decide to apply to be a chief resident?

I decided very early on to do it. First, I was very interested in being involved in resident and medical student education. Part of the job description is to be a facilitator between the residents and the faculty, so that was appealing to me as well, using my interpersonal skills within the system, in addition to patient and family interactions. You are an educator, politician, diplomat and facilitator. I wanted to continue to be involved with this very cool group of people and continue my training with some amazing faculty members.

How was your chief residency year different from your first year as a resident?

It was dramatically different from the first year. I was in a role of an attending physician and working with first-year residents without truly being that far from being in that position myself. I had a lot more confidence, but at the same time, a lot less experience than a seasoned faculty member. That made it scary, but in a very different way than the first year. I wondered if I knew enough to actually teach, as opposed to, "Do I know enough to not be a truly miserable failure as a doctor?"

What was memorable about your year as a chief resident?

There were several residents who had personal crises, and I ended up being very involved for all three of them, both being a support person within the residency, and also literally helping them change their schedules and their sets of expectations so they could continue to be residents. One had a death in the family, one had a major psychiatric issue with a family member and one was going through a divorce. It sort of mirrored patient care in a way, in that I was helping to facilitate people going through difficult periods and continuing to move forward with their own education and goals, which sort of mirrors being there in a patient crisis and altering treatment when life throws the patient a curveball.

One of the things that is appealing about family medicine is that because it is so broad, there are so many social issues that add to the medical complexity. It is very much about problem-solving skills, and the chief residency was problem-solving plus how to balance being a clinician with being a teacher/mentor.

I also helped design a major overhaul of the residency curriculum. The discussion of the ideas of what was going to happen took place in my third year, and the implementation itself happened in my chief year, and it was extremely exciting and challenging to be directly involved in the planning and implementation.

Who were your mentors during your residency?

Dr. Eric Walsh, for sure. He exemplified the passion for people and stories, which is what I love most about practicing medicine. He also has a true skill in conveying that passion and helping other people to remain inspired and excited. He is a fabulous doctor. For him, it is truly about stories and people, and his patients love him and his residents love him.

Also, Dr. Scott Fields, who is the chair of the program. He has a very, very different style than I do. It was rewarding to go work with him and to sort of see how a completely different style and personality type can be equally effective with patients. He is very passionate about teaching and very passionate about residents. He is a blunt, tell-it-like-it-is person, a do-not-soften-it-up kind of guy. It is easy to inadvertently be too nice when it could be damaging to the medical care of patients, and he was fantastic in teaching how to find the right balance in conveying harsh and difficult patient care messages in a very clear way without being unkind. He demonstrates that very well. My normal style is to soften around the edges and to put kindness at a higher value than clarity, and that is not always the right thing to do.

How did you balance your residency and your personal life?

It was easier, I think, for me to retain friendships because I am single and I do not have children. I was very impressed and amazed with some of my peers who maintained marriages and also were parents while sometimes working upwards of 100 hours a week — the ACGME duty hour standards came into effect after my second year. I cannot imagine how difficult that would be. I look on it that I had it easy during residency. It was hard balancing getting enough sleep, enough time for friends, and to find time for exercise, but I felt like I had the right balance.

What advice would you give to medical school graduates?

I would invite them to find mentors and, number two, to make a strong effort to check in with themselves periodically about where they are in the inspiration and burnout spectrum, and to make sure that they periodically find ways to inspire themselves. The worst thing that can happen is for the exhaustion to really start to dampen your soul. Burnout makes the practice of medicine mechanical, where inspiration makes it really magical and special. Making sure you do not fall too far in the burnout phase of the spectrum is one of the biggest challenges of internship.

What does medicine do well and what needs to be improved?

In terms of basic prolongation of life, after having the opportunity to practice medicine in Kenya and watching people die of tetanus, it is very evident how preventive medicine and immunizations and early intervention with active disease processes promote health. For people who have insurance and access, we do a decent basic job.

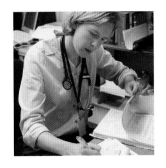 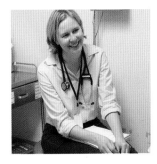 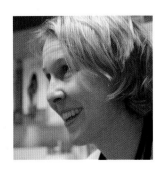

"FAMILY MEDICINE IS ABOUT WORKING WITH PATIENTS AS PEOPLE INTERACTING WITHIN THE CONTEXT OF THEIR FAMILIES AND COMMUNITIES."

However, given our resources, we do a pathetic job at getting healthy lifestyle messages out to patients and supporting, with dollars and energy, preventive types of programs and good mental health for uninsured and underinsured patients. So many people with insurance are underinsured, with limited access. We focus too much on expensive and highly technological end-of-life care, as opposed to doing prevention and health promotion.

I also think there is a false belief in medicine and in our society that everything is curable with the right amount of research, work and the right drug. That really extends to this cultural attitude that death is somehow a failure of will and intelligent medical care. Western medicine really promotes that attitude, which is clearly ridiculous and unhealthy for all of us. Sometimes a good death is the right goal in medicine. Sometimes the tubes and shocks in a patient with minimal chances of survival and quality of life are a failure of true care for a suffering patient and family. Obviously, it takes excellent communication to sort out the best course, but I saw an awful lot of futile and expensive medical care and unrealistic expectations during my training.

What are your career goals?

I do not know! I have been thinking about getting a master's degree in public health and getting more involved with health policy, especially international health policy, although I am also very interested in domestic health care access issues.

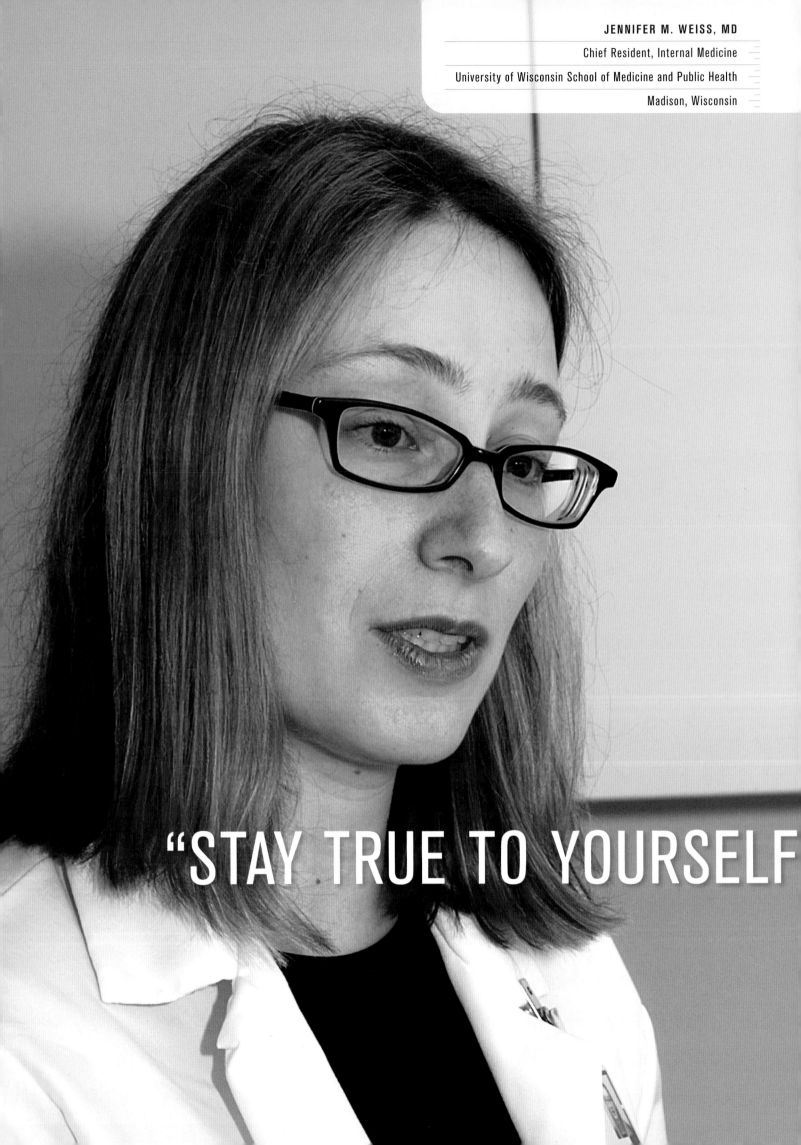

JENNIFER M. WEISS, MD

Chief Resident, Internal Medicine

University of Wisconsin School of Medicine and Public Health

Madison, Wisconsin

"STAY TRUE TO YOURSELF

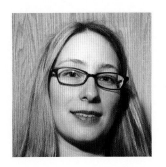

When Jennifer Weiss, MD, was growing up in Buffalo, New York, she had so many interests that she wasn't sure what she wanted to do for a career. However, a stint as a volunteer worker at a university health clinic pointed her toward medicine. Dr. Weiss earned an undergraduate degree in neurobiology at Cornell University, then completed medical school at the University of Rochester School of Medicine and Dentistry. While a medical student, she was given an award for best exemplifying the ideas of medicine.

She then did her residency in internal medicine at the University of Wisconsin School of Medicine and Public Health, where she served as chief resident in 2005–06. She also served as a resident representative to the Association of American Medical Colleges' Organization of Resident Representatives and mentored third-year medical students during their internal medicine clerkships.

Dr. Weiss is now enrolled in a fellowship program in gastroenterology at the University of Wisconsin. In her spare time, Dr. Weiss enjoys running, movies and spending time with her family and friends.

What made you decide to go into medicine?

Growing up I really had no idea what I wanted to do. I was just interested in so many different things. I thought about architecture for a little while, I thought about interior design, I thought about marine biology. In college I started in pre-med just because it seemed easy to do, in case I wanted to go to medical school, and get all the requirements done. I really loved it. I then wound up volunteering as a medical assistant at our University Health Service on the contraception, gynecology and sexuality services floor. I worked a lot with college-age women on pelvic exams, STD checks, doing a lot of educating on campus, and then dealt with some teenage pregnancies and really just got turned on to health care in general at that point. That's what made me actually go into medical school.

AND WHAT YOU BELIEVE IN."

Once I got into medical school, my background from college was neurobiology, so I thought about neurology quite a bit, but then I also thought about ob/gyn because of my interaction with the women's health services. When I did those rotations in medical school, it just didn't add up to everything I knew I wanted out of a career in medicine. So I kept my eyes open and looked around at all the different specialties and found that I loved general surgery and loved internal medicine, and really could not decide between the two. I wound up meeting with a bunch of the program directors at the University of Rochester in emergency medicine, general surgery and internal medicine, and the one thing that all three of them just suggested, after I told them why I liked both fields, was that I try an elective in gastroenterology. I did this elective in my fourth year of medical school and absolutely loved it. I decided this is what I'm going to do and the way to get there is through internal medicine, so that's what I ended up doing. I'm going to be completing my gastroenterology fellowship at the University of Wisconsin also.

I like the fact that you have a number of different organs involved in the gastrointestinal system. I like the idea of dealing with patients who might have malignancies, either colon cancer or pancreatic cancer — it was a combination of being able to deal with a whole bunch of different organs but yet still specialize and focus on one system. I really like doing the procedures, but at the same time I don't want to be in the operating room all day, and I really like the intellectual thinking about the differential diagnoses and seeing patients in clinic with continuity in that arena as well.

Why did you choose the University of Wisconsin for your residency?

I interviewed all over the country at tons of programs and after I interviewed here, I absolutely just loved it. It was my top choice by far. I loved the program director, I loved the residents I had met here, I really liked Madison. It just ultimately felt like the right place for me to be.

Do you remember what you felt like on the first day of your residency?

I was *very* excited but *very* nervous. I mean, you all of a sudden feel like, "Oh my God, people are actually going to listen to the orders that I write and the things that I say," whereas in medical school, you could always hide behind the intern or the senior resident and kind of defer things to them. It was just the sense of having a lot of responsibility and the fear of not knowing how much backup you're going to receive, and how much you're going to be out there on your own. And then it all turns out to be very nurturing and a very safe environment and there are tons of people who are there for your safety net, and as your resource, but you just don't know until you get there and see.

Does anything stand out from the first year of your residency?

I'm sure it's not just unique to my program, but I definitely was very surprised at how close the people in my intern class became, and just how close we still are and how we all would still do anything for each other if somebody needed it. That was just absolutely great. I'm very pleased at how amazing the attending physicians are at our institution, and how much support they give you to reach the goals that you've set for yourself. It just seems that everybody is there to help you get where you want to be, as well as help you become the best physician that you can be, and it was a very nice environment right from the start, and that definitely stood out to me.

How is the chief residency year different from and the same as your first year of residency?

Well, I think it's exactly the same in that you get thrown into a situation and you don't know what to expect and, again, you just start to feel nervous and excited all at once in the beginning. I think I knew how to handle teaching the residents and going through the lectures that we do every day, but there's a lot of administrative stuff that you kind of get sheltered from when you're a resident, and I was nervous about dealing with that and wasn't sure how I would handle it. There are a lot of challenges as far as being the kind of advisor that the residents feel they can come to, and just learning how to be the mediator, and learning how to take in the information, not pass any judgment, and then move on and get all sides of the story. I wasn't sure how good I would be at that, and how good I would be at being a resident advocate. At the same time, you have to be an advocate for the department and the administration, and help do what they need to get done for the residency program, but yet still protect the residents.

"I'VE LEARNED HOW TO PUSH MYSELF TO MY LIMITS."

The chief residency year is an extra year in your program. What made you decide to take the position instead of going straight to your fellowship?

When I was in medical school, I was really wowed by the chief residents in internal medicine because they, at every program, typically run all of the teaching conferences. It just seemed that they had an extensive knowledge base, they knew how to incorporate their knowledge into patient care, and they're great teachers. I've always been interested in teaching and always knew I wanted to stay at an academic center, so doing a chief residency year just kind of fell into what my overall plans were. I always thought that I was going to at least apply for it. Whether or not I got it — I wasn't sure until they told us. But I definitely want to stay at an academic institution, so doing an extra year where I hone my teaching skills, as well as hone some administrative skills, was very important for me. I'm definitely thinking about pursuing a position as a residency program director at some point, and so being a chief resident gave me great insight into whether or not that's something I want to pursue.

How do you feel you've grown both personally and professionally since you've started your residency?

I've definitely learned how to handle stress a lot better, I think. I definitely learned what my limitations are and when I need to ask for help, as well as learning who to go to when I do need help. I've also learned how to push myself to my limits and maybe not go for help so quickly. In medical school, you do a lot of just asking your resident, asking your intern, and they provide the answer for you, but you don't necessarily go and investigate and look a bunch of stuff up on your own, and I think I've gotten a lot better at that. It's definitely strengthened my sense of independence.

I've matured quite a bit during residency and I've learned a lot about working in a systems-based approach and working in a team and working with people of all different disciplines. These are skills that I didn't necessarily have as an intern but that grew throughout residency, and they are tested on a daily basis as a chief resident, when you're working with the nursing supervisors and the residents and the administration and pharmacy and trying to get everyone on the same page as far as policies with the ultimate goal of patient care in mind.

Is there any moment that stands out from your chief resident year?

Yes, every time a crisis comes up on the wards and I say to the intern who looks scared and the resident who doesn't know how to handle things "You know what? Why don't we step back and take a look at the situation. This is what we can do right now, this is what I can do for you later, let's call this consultant right now." I see the look in their eyes when they think, "Oh my God, I don't know if I'll be able to do that two years from now when I'm a senior resident." Just knowing how to handle the situation and being the one who is the calmest in a crisis definitely makes me feel good. When we do our teaching conferences and someone comes up to me afterwards and says "You know, I think I really actually understand pulmonary hypertension," it makes me feel good. It makes me feel like I'm helping in some way, and it solidifies what chief year actually means to me.

When did you start thinking of yourself as a doctor?

Somewhere about halfway through your intern year you start to all of a sudden feel, yeah, I am a doctor and I actually do know what I'm doing. Then about a month later, as you're just about to head into your second year and become a senior resident, you start to become extremely afraid that "Oh my God, now I'm going to be in charge of the team. I know I'm a doctor, but do I know enough to lead the new intern that's coming in a couple of months?" I think it's just a constant, continuous growth cycle where maybe about six or seven months into your position you start to feel a little bit comfortable, but then things switch up and you get new responsibilities a few months later and you feel like the new kid on the block again.

Who was most influential to you during your residency?

My program director, Dr. Bennett Vogelman, was the most influential. He just really seems to embody what a physician is in my mind, or what kind of a physician I want to become, as far as caring for his patients, having excellent relationships with his patients, continuing to practice on the wards and in his clinic, and always having his door open and being there for the residents when they need to stop in and talk to someone. He's extremely involved in our residency program and is always supportive of the residents and always has their best interests in mind. As a chief resident, I work much more closely with him, and I *really* get to see firsthand how he goes to the administration and fights for the residents. He is always trying to hook people up with mentors and get them in the field that they want to be in, and I truly believe that he sees residency as a stepping stone in someone's career and tries to help people get to where they want to be.

What advice would you give to medical school graduates entering their residencies?

You need to go to a program where you're going to feel comfortable, where you feel like you're going to be able to blossom and grow into your own, and you need to go into a program where you think you're going have fun. It's really important to be able to come home and relax in order just to stay fresh every day when you go back in.

It is important to stay true to yourself and what you believe in and not to lose sight of the values and things that made you go into medicine in the first place. If you do start to feel burned out and start to feel like you've lost sight of that, then find a mentor within your program, someone you can talk to, someone who can reinvigorate you.

If you could change one thing in medicine what would that be?

There's just such a pressure on physicians to see so many patients in a day and I think it really takes away from the actual time you can spend with a patient, building your relationship, finding out more about him/her. We order so many tests because we don't have time to do a good physical exam, and we don't have time to sit and actually listen to the history that the patients are telling us, which may give us an answer before we go and order this thousand-dollar CT scan. I wish that we could go back to a time when we didn't have to see a patient in 15 minutes.

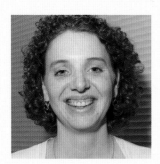

L anessa Bass, MD, says her mother, a nurse, was her inspiration to pursue a medical career. Dr. Bass grew up in the small town of Hawkins, Texas, about 100 miles east of Dallas. She earned a degree in genetics from Texas A&M University and briefly considered a career in genetic counseling before going back to her original career choice of pediatrics. Dr. Bass completed her medical degree at the University of Texas Medical Branch in Galveston in 2002 and then entered the pediatric residency program at the University of Arkansas for Medical Sciences. During her residency, Dr. Bass was named pediatric intern of the year, pediatric emergency department resident of the year, and pediatric resident teacher of the year. Following graduation in June 2006, she joined the pediatrics department at the University of Texas Health Center at Tyler.

In her spare time, Dr. Bass enjoys cardio boxing, reading and visiting her family in Hawkins.

Tell a little bit about yourself and why you decided to go into medicine.

My mom was a nurse. She finished nursing school when I was eight years old and I vividly remember her going through nursing school. She was a great student and put much effort into her studies. After she graduated, I would go with her to the hospital, even during some of her night shifts. I think being exposed to the medical field, and especially the care of patients, probably directed me to medicine. She definitely was my first teacher on the professionalism of medicine. She also was the one that told me to become a doctor. She passed away when I was 16, so I'm not, as an adult, able to ask her why a physician, but it stuck with me.

"I knew that I wanted

When I went to start my undergraduate work at Texas A&M, my world got broadened a lot. I learned about many different professions that I didn't get exposed to growing up in a small town. I then started thinking about other professions. I majored in genetics and I toyed around with the idea of going to graduate school to do genetic counseling. However, ultimately, I always came back to wanting to be a pediatrician. You can give such varied care, being a physician, and the interaction that you have with the patients you can't beat.

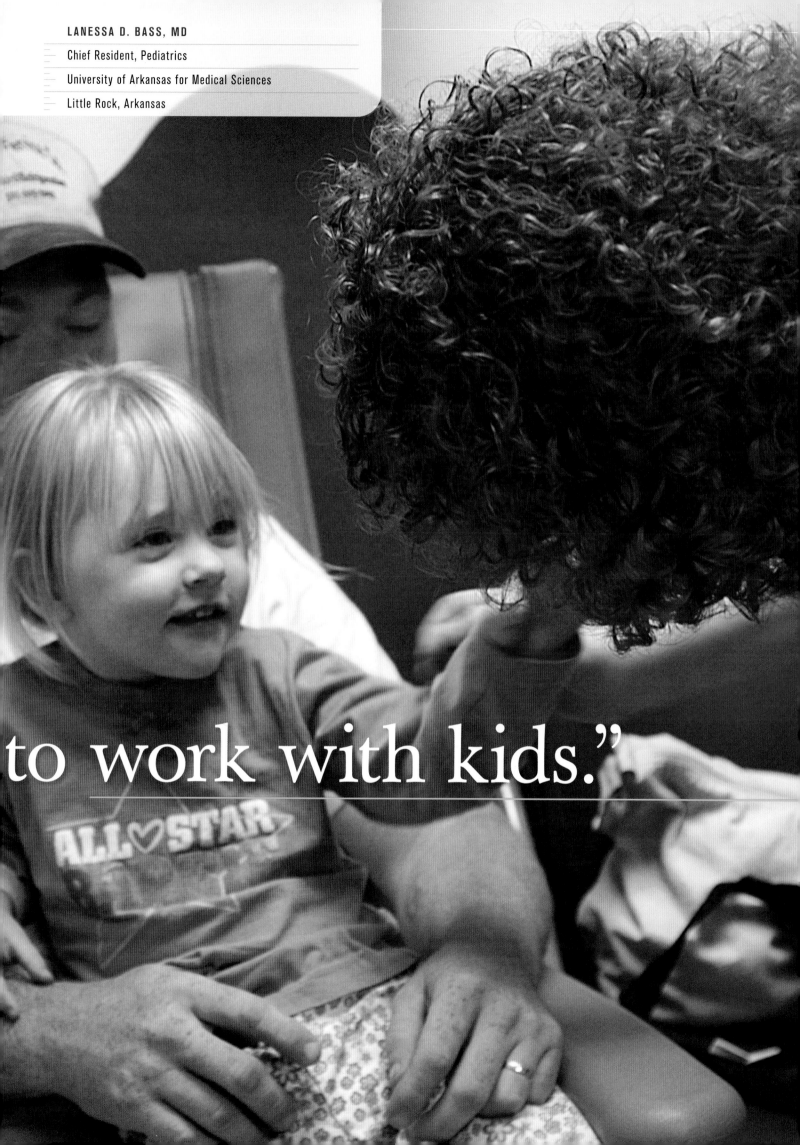

LANESSA D. BASS, MD

Chief Resident, Pediatrics

University of Arkansas for Medical Sciences

Little Rock, Arkansas

to work with kids."

Why did you choose pediatrics as a specialty?

Well, that was an easier decision. The hard decision was deciding — and I guess "hard" is not the right word — but the bigger decision was whether I was going to go to medical school or was I going to go to graduate school. But once I made the decision to go to medical school, I knew that I wanted to work with kids. From the very beginning of my first year at UTMB, I surrounded myself and exposed myself to the pediatric faculty there. I would say there are two types of medical students. One that will decide during their third or fourth year what residency they want to do; and others that knew from the very moment they walked into school. I definitely was the latter. I wanted to be a general pediatrician and never really wavered from that.

What do you remember about the first day of your residency?

I started out in the emergency room as an intern, and I remember walking into the emergency room — I can't remember if I wore my white coat or not; I think I probably did — and I noticed on the ER board it said July 1. On one of the clocks down the hall it said July 1. Everywhere I looked, it was reminding me that it was my first day of internship. I also, interestingly, noticed on the ER board that it said "ER Coordinator" and there was a person's name, "Nessa" underneath it, which is my nickname [laughs]. And I was, like, wait a minute, I'm not supposed to start out as coordinator. You know, I'm *just* an intern. But I found out that there was a Vanessa that worked there, who was a nurse [laughs].

I think most interns go to bed on June 30th wondering what they're going to be exposed to that first day and even throughout residency. You wonder if you're ever going to be in a situation where you feel that you're in over your head.

That first day stands out very clearly, and the other moment that stands out just as clearly was in the intensive care nursery. It was my second or third day in the unit. We had a 26-week preemie that was delivered, and the attending had to go to another delivery immediately. She said, "You need to get this baby stabilized and write the orders." That seemed pretty overwhelming at first, to have to write orders on an 800-gram infant, including drips and ventilator settings. However, I was able to do it, and I am happy to say that the baby did well and went home several months later. That's probably where I made that mental transition to making decisions quickly without looking for somebody else to back me up. That's when I think that I truly became, in my own mind, a physician.

Were you confident when you started your residency that you would learn all that you needed to know to become a physician in independent practice?

Yes. Enough people have gone through residency and have become confident, practicing physicians. You have to trust in the history behind the training system and trust in the residency program that you're training at. Now, there were times that, yeah, I was concerned with what might walk through the door, because kids can get sick pretty quickly. But did I feel like I would be exposed to a variety of things, have the backup to give great care to those kids, and then come out on the end having learned a lot? Yes, definitely. I think that's a testament to the training system that we have currently — if you go into training, really learn from the patients, learn from your faculty, read, work hard, you're going to become a good physician in the end.

What made you decide to become a chief resident?

In our program, in about October of our second year, our program director, our chairman of the department and current chiefs all sit down and talk about second-year residents that they think would be good chief residents. They decide on the first two that they would like to ask. The program director, generally the person that recruited you to the program, then officially offers you the position. How could you say no? Before I accepted, though, I promised myself that I would fight for the residents — not necessarily fight — but always be the resident advocate in that role. Plus, when I asked my family, they said, "When you are asked to serve, you serve!"

Describe a typical day as a chief resident.

It's different than residency itself; it's much more administrative. Misty Leigh [the other chief resident] and I are the direct managers of approximately 76 residents in our program. The largest job responsibility is scheduling month-to-month and then the yearly schedule. We also recruit for the incoming intern class. We handle conflicts among residents, residents and staff and residents and faculty. Luckily, we also continue to serve in a clinical role. At our program, chief residents are instructors, so we've moved into junior faculty positions. We attend on our inpatient service, in our emergency room and then we also attend either in our general pediatrics clinic or in the faculty clinic here. This advancement to the attending level may be one of the most beneficial parts of the chief residency year. For me it was another big transition point.

What moments as a chief resident have been particularly meaningful?

As a whole, it's when there's something that you've worked on, or the previous chiefs have worked on that you've continued, and you're starting to see the fruits of it. This year we had plans for a new resident lounge. That has been in the process for about a year and a half now, and we're starting to see the fruits of that. It's good because you're seeing the improvement and the stamp that you're leaving. Our program director told us that chief residents are generally remembered for two to three things that they accomplish during their year. He said if we can find our two or three things, then we're doing well.

Who has been the most influential or helpful to you in your residency?

I would say, professionally and personally, [former program director] Dr. Gordon Schutze has been the most influential. When I interviewed for residency, I could tell he really put his heart and soul into his residency program. But he also put his family first. He's pushed that on the

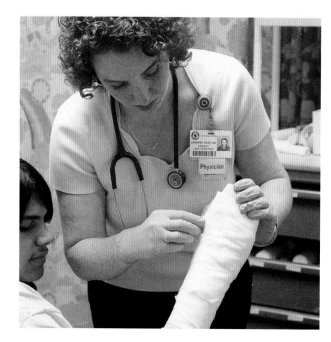
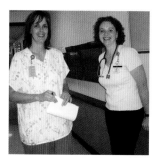
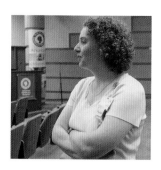

"IN PEDIATRICS, EVERY DAY THAT I SEE PATIENTS, THEY WILL MAKE ME SMILE AND LAUGH."

residents as well — that family comes before your profession and they are the ones you go home to. I have a lot of respect for that. Personally and professionally he's been a great mentor. There are many, many other people. I also found that one of my former chief residents, Becky Latch, has been very influential. She just carried herself with humor and kindness. I never thought she got flustered throughout her chief year. She might have, but she never showed it outwardly.

How do you think you've grown both as a physician and as a person since your residency started?

My ideal goal, when I went to medical school and then on to residency, was to continue to have compassion and patience with the families I worked with. Sometimes, with the stress and the hours of working, you lose a part of that. You lose some of the idealism.

I also am much more comfortable with the title here at the hospital. You know, I just went to a banquet recently for a previous scholarship I had received as an undergraduate. Several of the people kept saying, "Oh, it's Dr. Bass," and I still get embarrassed when people say that with some kind of awe. To me, it's my job. I'm proud of it, but it doesn't make me any better than another professional. My brother's a teacher, and other people outside of the school do not say, "Hey, that's Teacher Bass." And he is a great teacher!

But here in the hospital I feel very comfortable with that title. I don't take a second to answer it or a hesitation. There's just a confidence that this is the right place for me. This is the service that I can provide and where my energies make the most difference. Where are my talents going to be best utilized? Part of my talent is in working with families, motivating them. I don't mind hearing the routine questions that parents always have; I enjoy discussing that with them.

However, personally, what I'm still working on and hope to accomplish over the next six months is a balance. Residency requires a lot of you, requires a lot of hours. It requires you to sacrifice a lot, including family occasionally. Part of the reason I agreed to do the chief residency year was to bring a better balance to my life. Yes, you're going to do a lot for your patients, you're going to learn a lot, but you also need to give to your family, you need to give to yourself. To be successful, you have to have other avenues and other outlets. I'm still working on that. I think it's hard to adjust back down to a more normal speed of life. But I at least recognize the need to adjust.

What have you learned from the children that you treat?

You learn this zest for life, for having fun and not letting life get too serious. You see children with pretty horrific diseases and yet they still have this air about them — they just want to have fun, they just want to play. It keeps me young. In pediatrics, every day that I see a child, I am guaranteed to smile and laugh. I think it's healthy for a person to laugh every day, so luckily I go into a room and see a little infant's new skills and the parents' response to what they're learning — you can't help but laugh. This definitely lightens your load a little.

What are your plans after graduation?

I've accepted a position at an academic health center near my hometown, in Tyler, Texas. It actually is with the same hospital where my mom worked as a nurse and where I spent so many nights visiting her.

What is one thing that you think medicine does really well and one thing that could be improved?

The one thing medicine does really well is the technological advancements in care.

The one thing I would change is to try to advance our discussion on some of the ethics behind what we do. We're doing a lot with what we're able to do, but we haven't yet broached the subject of what we *should* do. Or maybe we've broached it but we haven't yet gone down the road much. Prolonging care, quality of life issues, medical futility — all this gets into pretty touchy political and ethical subjects, but I think it all needs to be advanced. If we continue just to go off of what we're able to do, but we never broach the subject of what we *should* with this technology, then your day-to-day clinical decisions are much harder. We don't have to come to a consensus immediately, but I think that the discussions need to start.

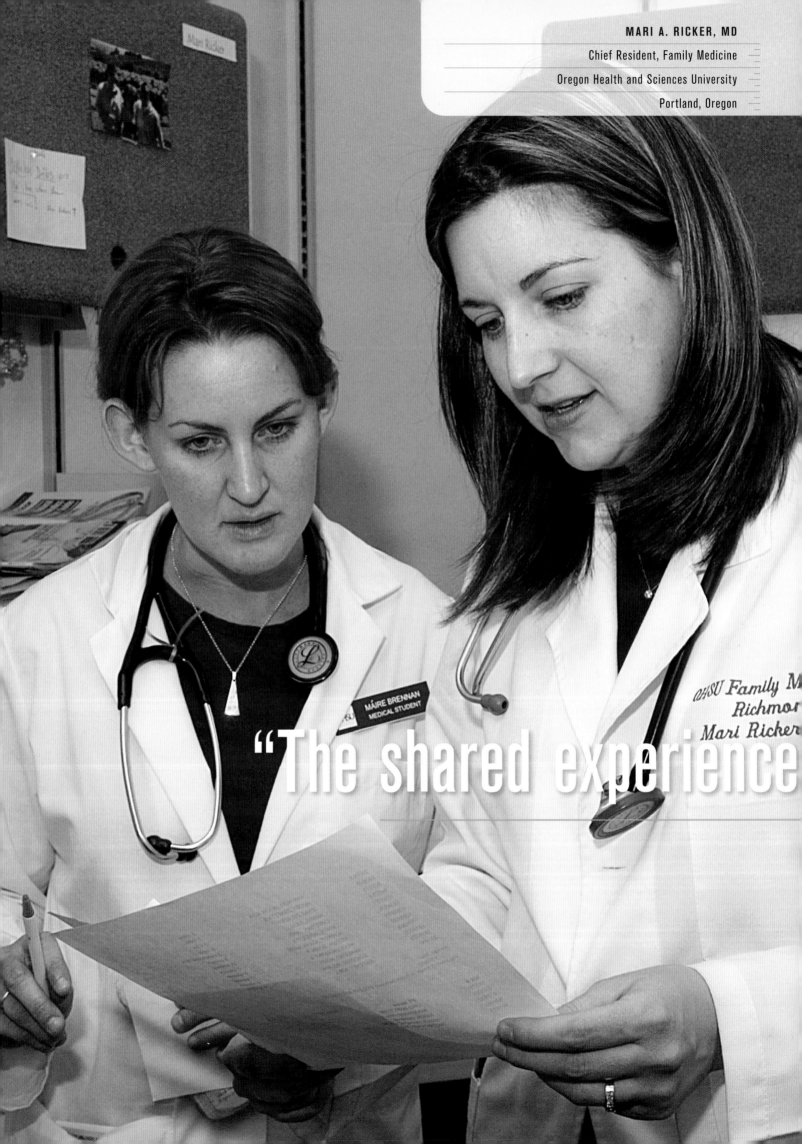

MARI A. RICKER, MD
Chief Resident, Family Medicine
Oregon Health and Sciences University
Portland, Oregon

"The shared experience

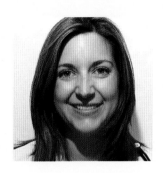

A s a young woman with a flair for science and math, Mari Ricker, MD, was encouraged to pursue a career in engineering or science. However, she found those areas did not satisfy her desire to teach and help other people. She realized that medicine would give her the mix of science and interaction with people that she wanted.

Dr. Ricker was born in England and raised in Arizona. She earned an undergraduate degree in biology from the University of Virginia and completed her medical degree at the University of Arizona. She served as chief resident in family medicine at Oregon Health and Sciences University in 2005–06. In her free time, Dr. Ricker enjoys spending time with her husband, a Spanish teacher and soccer coach, doing yoga, running, walking with her dog, knitting and skiing.

Why did you decide to become a physician?

I was interested in a lot of different things. My mom works for a theater company and my dad worked as a teacher for most of his life. My mom's dad, who lived in England, was a bacteriologist. There were so many things that I could see myself doing, and I liked all the science parts of engineering, but didn't like that there were so many things you didn't get to deal with — the personalities, conversations, families, things like that. Somehow, I came up with the idea that medicine would be right for me because it mixed science and people. Once I had decided that was my plan, I did some one-week internships with doctors in Phoenix during Christmas vacation. I was always drawn to family medicine because I liked the idea of looking at the person as a whole, integrated into their homes and families, and everything.

was the most important thing."

What was the first day of your residency like?

My first rotation was starting in the newborn intensive care unit, and I was absolutely terrified. There were these tiny little babies that were 27-weeks old, and I was petrified starting an internship, and on top of it, these babies were preemies. Over the course of that month I got more comfortable with the babies.

Every month my rotation was brand new, and I was trying to figure out a new age-set. I had this incredible anxiety before starting a rotation, like I was starting my internship all over again. More than the new age-set that I was getting to know, it was also the people, the systems, the expectations that seemed to stress me out. Going from tiny babies to the Veterans Administration population definitely was a shock.

I got most of my support from the 11 other interns in my class. We were, and are, incredibly close and now ten of us live within a square mile in Portland. The shared experience was the most important thing.

Does any moment from the first year stand out?

I had kind of a traumatic experience on New Year's Eve. I had gotten a needlestick from a patient in November, and nothing had come back yet, and they had just rechecked my blood for some tests, and I found out on New Year's Eve 2002 that I had contracted Hepatitis C. That was probably the bottom of my year. I was tired and exhausted and stressed and not sure if I was being a good doctor, and then I had this hit about my own health. I felt like I had been giving, giving, giving to people and this institution, and now I had contracted this disease. That was pretty traumatic to me. I ended up taking several days off and coming back to work. My program was so supportive through that experience, and my classmates were as well. One of my faculty searched down a hepatologist, and two or three months later I ended up clearing it from my blood. So I didn't, and shouldn't, have any long-term effects from it.

Did you feel confident that you would learn all you needed to know to become a physician in independent practice?

The first year I felt overwhelmed. Each month you are learning a whole new bag of a patient population and new set of diagnostics. I think it took an entire year for me to feel like it was coming together, all those pieces I had been learning bit by bit. You just get through this year, just show up and keep going. I had to go on faith that it would come together.

We had one day off between intern year and second year, and all of us interns went out to the coast and rented a house for a night and kind of debriefed and talked about our emotions and the things that had happened. We sat around and checked in on the best moment of the year and the worst moment of the year. The last thing we talked about was the things we were grieving that year. People had so many things, from patients to relationships with family members, to parts of themselves that had gone away.

There are things that I identify as being part of my personality that I haven't had time to focus on, things that I formerly enjoyed doing. I enjoyed dancing and keeping in touch with my friends, and I really identify myself as having a gregarious and joyful personality — and toward the end of the year I didn't even feel like myself. I felt like that had been taken away.

What is your chief residency year like?

Ours is a bit different. Three of the residents act as clinic chiefs, but I am doing a chief residency as a fourth year.

I started thinking about applying as a chief resident somewhere in my intern year. I really enjoy the leadership role and the biggest thing, the thing that I thought would be the best fit for me, is the interpersonal relationship with the residents. I am finding that those parts that I thought would be really easy have been the most challenging for me. The other parts of the chief resident year are getting to work more closely with the faculty and the leadership and the department.

I've definitely enjoyed it. I think the surprising thing is that the things I thought would come easily have been more challenging. When I was a first-, second-, or third-year resident, I had the 11 other residents to bounce things off of, but now I get brought all the negative things, like this-isn't-going-well, someone-is-sick but I don't have the positive feedback where you all go through the same thing.

How have you grown as a person and doctor?

The way you change from the beginning of your internship to the end of your third year is astronomical. You spend three years putting it together clinically and figuring out what sort of physician you are going to be and figuring out what sort of boundaries you are going to have with patients. I am an emotional person and I get drawn into patients' stories. You need to set up those healthy boundaries with patients who want you to cross over and get too involved or who try to manipulate you. I worked with a pretty challenging population that had high needs. Over the past six months I have seen myself change so much in the transition from being a resident to junior faculty, and also seeing from a faculty perspective the needs of the department and how it is challenging to manage 36 residents and keep the curriculum up.

Are there any moments that have been particularly meaningful this year?

I think over the past couple of weeks we've had some tragedies among the residents. I feel like it's been an honor to sit in with the residents. Last week we had a situation where we spent a half hour trying how to figure out how to support a resident who was going through a tough time. I felt honored that they allowed me to be there and try to rally around this resident.

What advice would you give to medical school graduates starting their residencies?

To not be too hard on themselves. I often see them trying to figure it all out themselves and feeling really frustrated when they don't have all the skills they expect to have. It just takes time and repetition and patience.

If you could change one thing in medicine, what would that be?

If I could change one thing it would be to create an openness to change the paradigm about how we study. There are a lot of things we don't study very well because of this paradigm we have set up, like the connection between the body and the mind. I would hope that medicine as a profession could figure out a way to incorporate that in our culture. In family medicine we take care of a lot of different ailments that are completely connected with anxiety and depression; things like asthma and hypertension are affected by stressors.

What are your plans after your residency?

I took a job as faculty at a community family medicine program here in Portland at Providence Milwaukie Hospital. I have really enjoyed teaching the medical students. I'm also pregnant, so I will have lots of new things going on this year!

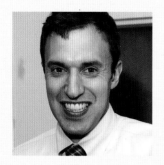

T homas Renaud, MD, always knew that he wanted to work with children. As a college undergraduate and medical student at the University of Vermont, Dr. Renaud launched a meal preparation program at a local Ronald McDonald House, coached a soccer team and organized groups of medical students to give presentations at elementary schools. A love of science — he majored in biology and philosophy — drew him to medical school, where a rotation in pediatrics clinched his decision to become a pediatrician.

Dr. Renaud, who is married, unwinds from his job by going to movies and restaurants with his wife, also a pediatrician. Following graduation from his residency program, Dr. Renaud began a hematology-oncology fellowship.

Why did you decide to go into medicine?

I double-majored in biology and philosophy, thinking that I would go into biological research, the PhD track. I certainly enjoyed the science aspect of it but kind of missed out on the people interaction. So I started looking for what else I should do, and a couple of friends suggested medicine. I looked into it and talked to my family doctor quite a bit, spent some time in the local hospital, and really saw a bit of how things worked and what people did, and it just kind of clicked with me. So that is what sort of brought me into medicine initially.

"You learn a lot about taking

Why did you choose pediatrics as a specialty?

Well, there are a few pieces to it. I have always been involved with kids for as long as I can remember. I worked at summer camps throughout high school and college and coached a bunch of soccer teams and groups like that. Kids have always been a lot of fun for me. I just enjoy spending time with them and always find them refreshing. Once I got to know the different services during my clinical core year in medical school — pediatrics, surgery, all those sorts of things — I really grew to enjoy pediatricians. They seemed obviously intelligent and motivated and all that you want in your colleagues, but also interested in the bigger picture when it comes to kids — interested in the family, how they are viewing either the health of their child or the illness that their kid might have, and also interested a bit more broadly in society. By the nature of what we do, pediatricians are interested in epidemiology and a population-based approach to medicine. That is very interesting for me, also.

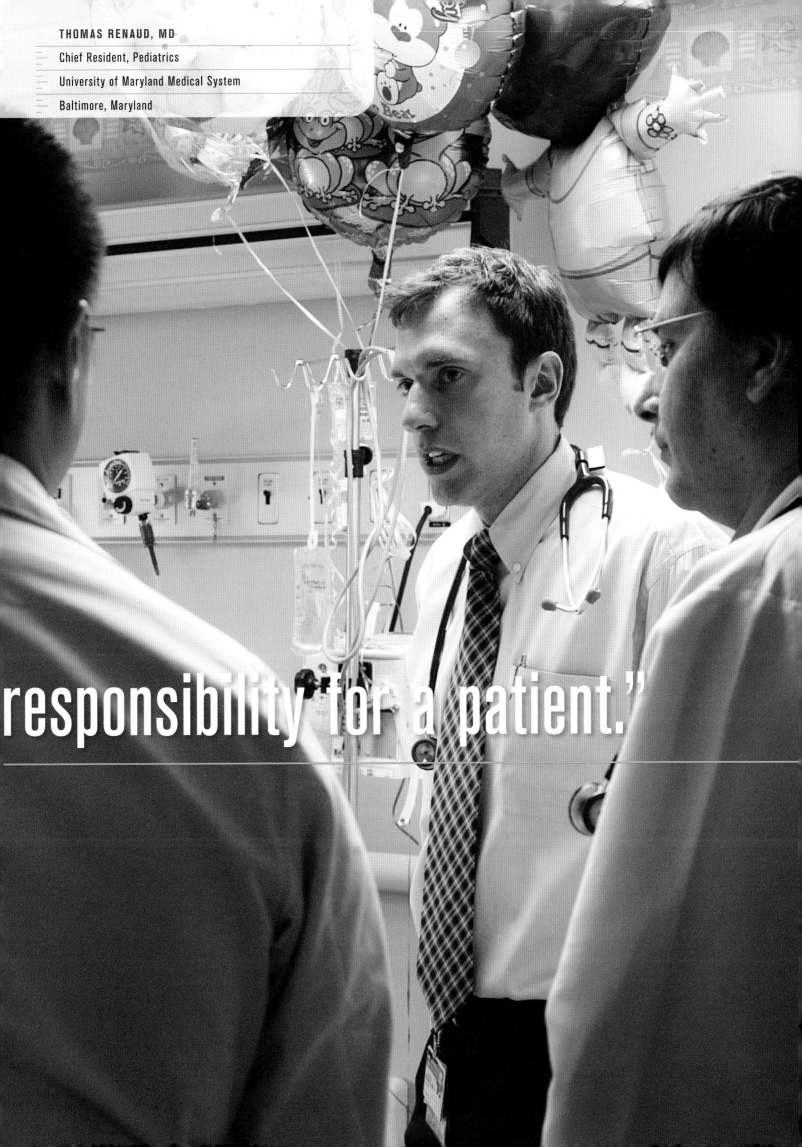

THOMAS RENAUD, MD

Chief Resident, Pediatrics

University of Maryland Medical System

Baltimore, Maryland

responsibility for a patient."

Why did you decide to go to the University of Maryland for your residency?

As I was doing a lot of interviews, I figured out I wanted a medium-sized academic program. That shortened my list a fair amount, and ultimately it came down to the people that I met here. The residency director here is wonderful, Dr. Carol Carraccio, and the residents that I met were just good people; they were warm, intelligent, caring people, and it just seemed like a good place to work. It seemed like they enjoyed each other, they supported each other, and that really drew me in.

It is a three-year program. It has an extra year of chief residency beyond that. I am in a bit of an unusual situation. The program decided to start two of us in our chief year during our third year, so we are both doing an extra year, but each of us spent half of our third year being chiefs and half being residents and half of our fourth year doing chief.

Do you remember what you were feeling when you started your residency?

It was pretty scary [laughs]. You kind of walk in and feel like, "Well, I just finished being a medical student and all of a sudden right now they expect me to be a doctor." You do not quite realize that it is a much more subtle and long-term process than that. You kind of walk in your first day, thinking, "Oh my God, they are going to expect me to know everything and I do not feel like I know anything." But it is much slower than that. I think that there is a lot of trepidation, there is a lot of worry about, "Oh, no, am I going to hurt patients because I do not know anything? Am I going to look stupid because I do not know anything?" But that is mostly misperception.

What stands out from your first year?

One of the big things that stood out for me was a patient that I took care of who was diagnosed with a brain tumor. I saw her in the ER when she was initially admitted. She had come from another country to get care here, and I saw her in the ER and evaluated her, and you could tell right away that something pretty significant was going on. And I continued to follow her. I had her for a month when I was on the floor, and I had her for a little bit of time in the ICU, so just by sheer chance I took care of her on many services and got to know the family very, very well. Unfortunately, she had a very difficult-to-treat tumor, and she passed away late in my first year. That was really tough. I had taken care of her many times; I really knew her very well. You learn a lot from that. You learn that you get attached to folks, and that can be extremely difficult when things do not go well. That was a big learning experience for me.

You learn a lot about taking responsibility for patients — making sure that the next person who takes care of them is following up on this lab or that scan or whatever, and you learn how important it is to do all those little things, to make sure all those things get passed on and make sure everyone else is aware of them.

How is your chief residency year different from and the same as your earlier years of residency?

Most of it is pretty different. You do very little patient care as a chief resident. Here we do one afternoon a week of our continuity clinic, so we see eight outpatients for one afternoon a week. Other than that, you do not do very much patient care; it is almost purely an administrative job at this institution. A lot of the job is essentially personnel management — creating schedules for people, coordinating different services. One of the big differences is that you get a lot of interaction with both residents and the faculty, and you get a much broader view of what goes on in a residency program. It is funny: you are hearing things from both sides; you are hearing residents looking for things that they want to make the residency program better, you are hearing from faculty how they want to make the residency program better. Sometimes they are the same things and sometimes they are not. It is always very interesting to see the different perspective that people have based on where they are in their training.

As a chief resident, you sort of have responsibility for the mental health of your residents. Residency is not easy. You are asking people to work overnight and to work on weekends and be away from their families a lot, so you have to really keep that in mind.

The duty-hour standards have changed things. Whereas you used to just plug people into a floor schedule, now there are all sorts of changes you have to make during a month, and changes in clinics and changes in schedule, all based on the 80-hour workweek. It has changed things dramatically.

In your residency, did you feel confident that you would learn all that you needed to know to become a competent physician?

I did all along. In my first year, that was based purely on faith, assuming and hoping that it would happen, but then, as I sort of progressed on in my years, I started to realize, "Wow, that patient — I really made all the decisions. That kid — I knew how to take care of him." You gain that confidence with more and more complicated patients. You certainly get there. It is hard to see for sure that it will happen in the beginning, so some of it is just believing that it will.

How have you grown, both as a physician and as a person, since the first year of your residency?

I have certainly grown a lot as both. I guess, as a physician, it is just a remarkable change that you go through from early in your internship to late in your third year. Early in your internship, you often feel lost at sea. You often feel like you are not even sure of the right questions to ask. It is very disconcerting; you feel like you went to four years of medical school and you are not quite sure why sometimes [laughs]. But then you develop a lot more confidence, you learn you do have a good knowledge base and you learn how to use it as a resident, basically. There is a lot of growth in terms of confidence, for sure. I mean, I feel vastly more confident than I did when I came in as an intern. I feel like I have a skill to offer patients, that I can provide them some help and some benefit, whereas as an intern, you do not. I am starting to feel like all the hard work I have done so far is worth it, that I can see where I am going and that I will be able to do this in the future.

Certainly my career in medicine and my residency have helped me to grow as a person … but I think that a lot of my growth has occurred because of events outside of my residency program. Close to two years ago now, my wife's brother passed away very suddenly of complications from mononucleosis. That has really been the defining event of the last couple years of my life, and it has really changed how I look at life.

He was 20 at the time. Mononucleosis is one of those common illnesses that we treat in pediatrics all the time. Kids usually do fine with it. It was an incredibly traumatic event for us. Also, as doctors, we thought, "Well, gosh, did everyone do everything they should have? Were there mistakes made anywhere? What if we had talked to them?" All these things go through your head, which, of course, are irrational and not hopeful, but, because of how we learn to do medicine and how we learn to think about things, you always think about that. For a long time afterward, it brought up a lot of emotion treating kids who were diagnosed with mononucleosis or whom I suspected of it. That has been a major factor in my life, and I am still learning things from it, and I will continue to learn things from it for the rest of my life.

How do you balance your personal life with your professional life?

That is extremely challenging. My wife is also a pediatric resident; she is going to graduate this year, too. The good side of that is that she always understands that when I have call, I cannot get out of it; I cannot just take the night off. That is extremely helpful. The downside is that she also works a lot, so we see each other that much less. We are very careful to make sure that we make time for each other and make a real effort to be good to each other. My wife and I both enjoy films. We are close to DC; so we visit museums whenever we can. There are a lot of wonderful restaurants around here; we will go out to have some time to ourselves and not worry about work and just enjoy being together. We decided to wait to have children until after our residency is done. That was a tough decision to make, but we felt we would not have enough time to give our child, or children, the energy that they deserved.

Who has been influential to you during your residency?

The person who stands out for me is Dr. Neil Grossman, who is one of two hematology-oncology attendings here. He has been a major figure in my education as a resident and obviously also an important person in determining my future career in hematology-oncology. Like a lot of hematology-oncology doctors, he does wonderful patient care, takes incredible care of his patients, tends to everything, really makes them feel like there is someone who is going to make everything okay. That is an important characteristic that I want to have. He is also very funny; he jokes a lot with the residents, and he also jokes a lot with the parents when it is appropriate. That is incredibly important. Academic medicine can be a very serious field because people feel like this is life and death every day, and you do not fool around with that. But people like Dr. Grossman realize that is no way to live.

Do any moments from your chief residency year stand out?

There were a couple of moments that I will not forget. When you are the chief resident, you hear a lot of bad news — you know, when residents have a family emergency and need to miss time. There have been deaths of a couple of family members of people I am pretty close to in the residency. You are the first business call they make. They speak to their families and make those connections, but then the next thing they have to do is say, "I am not going to be at work for the next week." That has been something that I did not anticipate before starting as a chief resident, and it has been particularly hard.

What have you learned from the children you care for?

An incredible amount [laughs]. If I were to pick one thing, it is that you should never give up. You never know when things are going to take a turn for the better, and you never know what is going to happen, so you just have to keep hoping and keep working towards what you want and what you hope to have happen.

There are kids who have had tumors that should not have been able to be treated, but they got better. A two-year-old girl who had a congenital heart disease was in the intensive care unit and had cardiac arrests and was extraordinarily sick. A year later she was sitting up, doing fairly developmentally appropriate things: laughing and scribbling with some crayons. That is why we do this. There are plenty of kids who will not make it but there sure are a lot of kids who will. That is why we are here.

What advice would you give to medical school graduates just starting their residencies?

I would tell them to go on a nice vacation before they start. After they start, I would tell them to relax, it is going to be okay. A lot of that fear and trepidation is appropriate; it shows that you are interested in taking care of your patients. But the reality is that you are getting a lot of supervision when you start. People are there to help you. The weight of the world is not on your shoulders at that point.

What is one thing that you think can be improved in medicine, as well as one thing that medicine does particularly well?

One of the more important things in medicine that could be changed is the undergraduate medical education. You get steeped in this myriad of knowledge from so many different areas: histology, pathology, biochemistry, genetics. In some ways, we have kind of lost sight of the bigger picture. You are trying to learn so many specific pieces of information that you lose your perspective of the bigger picture and where all these things tie in. I think there is a certain amount of information that is taught in the basic sciences that is not necessary.

In this country, we have learned a tremendous amount, and we have learned how to treat an incredible number of diseases that we did not even know anything about, just 20 years ago. I think that the explosion of knowledge in the field is incredibly exciting.

BRANDI W. TRAMMELL, MD

Chief Resident, Obstetrics and Gynecology

Yale-New Haven Medical Center

New Haven, Connecticut

"Obstetrics is something

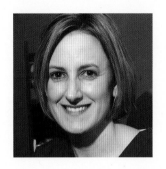

Brandi W. Trammell, MD, *always wanted to be a physician, but she wasn't sure which specialty she wanted to practice. After graduating from Auburn University in Montgomery, Alabama, with a degree in physical science, Dr. Trammell entered the University of South Alabama College of Medicine with thoughts of becoming either a pediatrician or a surgeon. However, after a rotation in obstetrics and gynecology, she found her calling. She completed the first two years of her residency at the University of South Alabama and then transferred to the ob/gyn residency program at Yale-New Haven Medical Center for the remainder of her residency.*

Dr. Trammell is married to an attorney. In their free time, Dr. Trammell and her husband enjoy snow and water skiing, biking and going to movies.

Why did you decide to go into medicine and what drew you to obstetrics and gynecology?

Even as a child, I remember wanting to be a doctor. I still vividly recall visits to my family physician, Dr. Morris, as a child when I was sick. Certainly no child enjoys being ill, but I did enjoy seeing him. He would sit me on his doctor stool and let me listen to my heartbeat with his stethoscope. I admired him a great deal and looked forward to the day when I would be a "grown-up" and could be a doctor.

that chooses you."

I'm the first physician in my family. I went to college at Auburn University at Montgomery and then attended medical school at the University of South Alabama College of Medicine in Mobile, Alabama. When I entered medical school, I planned on becoming a pediatrician or surgeon. However, things changed while rotating through the obstetrics and gynecology clerkship during my third year of medical school. I'm not sure that I would say that I chose obstetrics and gynecology. I feel that obstetrics and gynecology is something that chooses you, or me in this case. I found that I loved taking care of female patients. Ob/gyn is a wonderful specialty that allows you to take care of women throughout the various stages of their lives. You deliver their children during their reproductive years. Then, later in life, you are there to manage their gynecologic needs. The continuity of care is amazing. For me that's the perfect thing. Ob/gyn is also a dynamic specialty: you never know what each new day will bring.

What was the first day of your residency like?

I remember being excited and a little nervous. Starting residency marked the beginning of a new phase in my life and career. I began my first day at 6:30 a.m. I was assigned to be the first resident from my class, and residency program for that matter, to rotate at an outside hospital called The Mobile Infirmary Medical Center in Mobile, Alabama. The term *outside hospital* simply refers to any hospital which is not the primary place of residency training. I arrived and greeted the patient who was scheduled for a hysterectomy that morning. I remember assisting the attending physician with the surgery and enjoying every minute.

Did you feel confident that you would learn all you needed to know to become a doctor in independent practice?

Yes and no. I was confident in my abilities. However, it's a bit scary when you are called "doctor" for the first time. While being called a doctor is a wonderful privilege, the title carries tremendous responsibility and expectation. Although you are called doctor the day after graduating from medical school, it takes years of training before a young physician is ready to practice independently.

Are there any moments that stand out from your first year?

First year, no. Second year, yes. While on a high-risk obstetrics rotation, I had the pleasure of caring for a woman expecting twins with preterm premature ruptured membranes. She was on my service for many weeks. I rounded on her twice a day. Over the course of her hospitalization, we got to know each other quite well. Around 23 weeks she went into labor. A cesarean section was performed and twin baby girls were delivered and transferred to the neonatal intensive care unit. One night during the following week, one of the twins passed away. I was working at the hospital that night and happened to walk to the NICU to check on the status of the twins as events unfolded. I will never forget that night. Watching any infant die is a painful experience. Watching a patient and her husband hold their daughter in their arms and say goodbye is a life changing experience. On a happier note, the second twin did well and eventually was discharged from the hospital after many months. A year later I was invited to her birthday party. Although I was unable to attend due to work obligations, I was honored to be invited.

What does it feel like to deliver babies?

To me, every birth is a miracle. Delivering babies is always fun. You never know what the delivery is going to be like. Some women are very stoic and don't make a sound. Other women are more expressive, meaning they scream. It is not uncommon to have family members cheering them on. Ultimately, we all want an uncomplicated delivery and a healthy baby.

What is your chief resident year like? How is it different from the earlier years of your residency?

The chief year is unlike any of the other residency years. It is the year when decisions are made about your final career path. Some choose to continue with their training by pursuing fellowships in a subspecialty. Others decide to remain generalists and enter private practice. As one of the administrative chief residents at Yale, the responsibility was tremendous. The administrative chief residents share the burden with the faculty of assuring that the residency program runs smoothly. Anytime there is a problem with call schedules, resident morale, residents needing time away from work, you name it; it's your job to take care of it.

The expectations are also much greater. As a chief, you run your respective service, whether it is gynecology, obstetrics or others. You are ultimately responsible. This is a far cry from being an intern, where you are expected to be unsure of yourself and need guidance from your upper residents. As a chief, you are expected to know everything that goes on and have a reason for why something did or did not happen.

"YOU NEVER KNOW WHAT THE DELIVERY'S GOING TO BE LIKE."

Have there been any moments from your chief resident year that have been especially meaningful?

I can't recall a specific event that stands out more than others. I was honored to be selected as an administrative chief resident by my fellow residents and faculty. In general, I think that the chief year is a year of reflection. I am thankful to all the wonderful physicians and residents that I have worked with over the past four years. Each one has impacted my life greatly. Whether it's an attending physician teaching me ways to improve my surgical technique or a resident laughing with me over lunch, each played an important role in my becoming a better person and physician. The bonds that you form with others who are in the trenches with you are unbreakable.

How do you feel that you've grown, both personally and as a doctor, since you started your residency?

I have grown in a number of ways. I am more educated and confident. I have learned what things are worth worrying about and what things aren't. I have learned to be professional, compassionate, and diplomatic. Most importantly, I have learned how to form friendly relationships with patients, colleagues and staff. Being able to relate to others is a must in the medical profession. As long as you can be positive, treat others with the same respect that you would demand and enjoy what you do, work is not simply a job. It becomes a passion. I love being an ob/gyn. I can't imagine doing anything else.

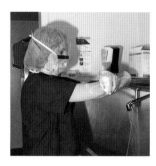
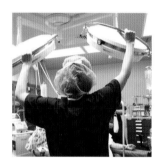
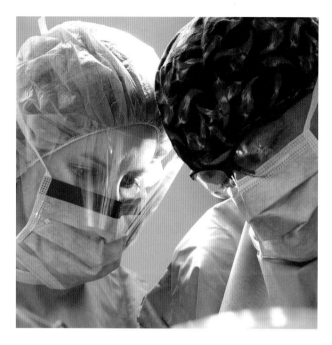

"MAKE SURE YOU PICK SOMETHING YOU LOVE."

Who has been the most influential or helpful to you during your residency?

Two gynecologic oncologists at Yale, Dr. Peter Schwartz and Dr. Thomas Rutherford, influenced me the most during residency. Both physicians are second to none. They are excellent surgeons, clinicians and people in general. Their patients respect and depend on them to make life-and-death decisions. The knowledge that I learned while on the gynecology oncology service at Yale is invaluable. Not only did I learn outstanding surgical technique or proficiency and how to manage critically ill patients, I also learned how to communicate with patients during difficult circumstances. I will consider my medical career a success if one day my patients think of me in the same regard.

What advice would you give to medical school graduates who are starting their residencies?

Most importantly, choose a specialty that you love. Many medical school students are choosing specialties based on average hours worked per week or medical-malpractice premium costs. They seem to have forgotten why they went into medicine in the first place. Hopefully, they chose medicine because they wanted to make a difference. At least, I would bet that is what they said during their medical school interview. They should know that all medical specialties require sacrifice. For me, I would rather spend twelve hours a day working in a profession that I love verses working eight hours a day in one that I settled for based on theoretical risks.

As an intern, it is easy to feel overwhelmed. Don't be. Your senior residents and faculty are always available and eager to help you. Ask them for help. Don't try to reinvent the wheel. Also, interns should accept criticism without taking it personally. Keep an open mind as you progress through residency. You will be a better physician for it. Also, treat those above and below you with the same respect. Learning to work as a team player is vital.

If you could change one thing in medicine, what would that be?

Access to health care continues to be a problem in the United States. We still see patients who present at term who have never received prenatal care. We continue to see patients who need operations for gynecologic indications who are uninsured and cannot afford the hospital costs. As a physician, I am frustrated by not being able to help all those in need.

What works well in medicine?

In general, the health care services in the United States are unsurpassed. People can present to the emergency room and receive the care that they need in an acute setting. They will receive the medications that they need, the emergency testing and imaging, the lifesaving surgery. They are treated and discharged home. There are definitely other places in the world where that type of care is not possible.

What are your career plans after you graduate?

I plan to enter private practice in Mobile, Alabama.

Is there anything else you'd like to say about your residency?

The entire process is one of maturing and learning. Not only do you obtain the knowledge needed to practice medicine, but also you learn a lot about yourself in the process. I remember hearing the statement "What does not kill you makes you stronger" throughout childhood. Residency exemplifies this statement. Residency, and ob/gyn in particular, reminds me of a roller coaster. It has its ups and downs and can be bumpy at times. Overall though, I have enjoyed the ride. I would like to especially thank the faculty, residents, and staff at Yale-New Haven Hospital for all their instruction, love, and support.

46   52   58   64

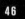

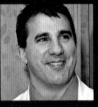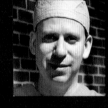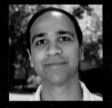

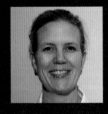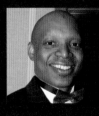

72   78   84

SURGEONS

"The thought processes go from 'I am doing things because I do not want to get in trouble' as a junior, to 'I am doing things because I want to do the case right' as a chief resident."

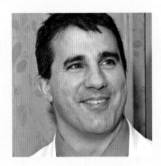

S hahab Abdessalam, MD, knew he wanted to be a doctor from the time he was a child. After receiving degrees in English and biology from Ohio State University, Dr. Abdessalam entered medical school at Ohio State and earned his medical degree in 1995. He then continued his education with residencies in surgery, surgical oncology and a fellowship in critical care medicine, all in preparation for his residency in pediatric surgery at Ohio State University, where he was chief resident in 2005–06. In 2000, Dr. Abdessalam was honored as the outstanding chief surgical resident at the University of Nebraska Medical Center, and in 2004 he was named surgical house officer of the year at Columbus Children's Hospital.

Dr. Abdessalam is married and has three children. An avid athlete, in his off-time he enjoys spending time with his family biking, golfing, hiking and skiing.

Why did you decide to become a physician?

I essentially always wanted to go into medicine. I was recently looking at a book report that I did in seventh grade. In the biography portion of the book report, I said I wanted to go into medicine and be a surgeon. That was always my objective. I saw medicine as a constant learning environment where there was always something new, and that really attracted me.

"Role models are

Being able to learn is one of the most unique things about being human and what makes us most alive. Medicine is therefore a profession that makes me feel most alive. On top of that, being able to help people to the point of bringing them back to life, altering a disease to prolong someone's life, or simply making their quality of life better gives a lot of purpose to my own life. So those were my biggest attractions to medicine.

As far as my choice of field within medicine, I liked the immediacy that surgery had, the impact that I could have right away. Also as a surgeon, I view myself as a physician who can operate. I did not want any limitations on what I could potentially do to help a patient. It was my original intention to do general surgery, but then I saw the limitations that general surgeons have put on themselves due to subspecialties. I liked the general aspect of general surgery — you can operate anywhere on the body and take care of the entire patient. When I was in med school I came into contact with oncology and really liked that aspect of medicine. I thought if I really wanted to make an impact, oncology seemed the place to do it. It has the complexities of

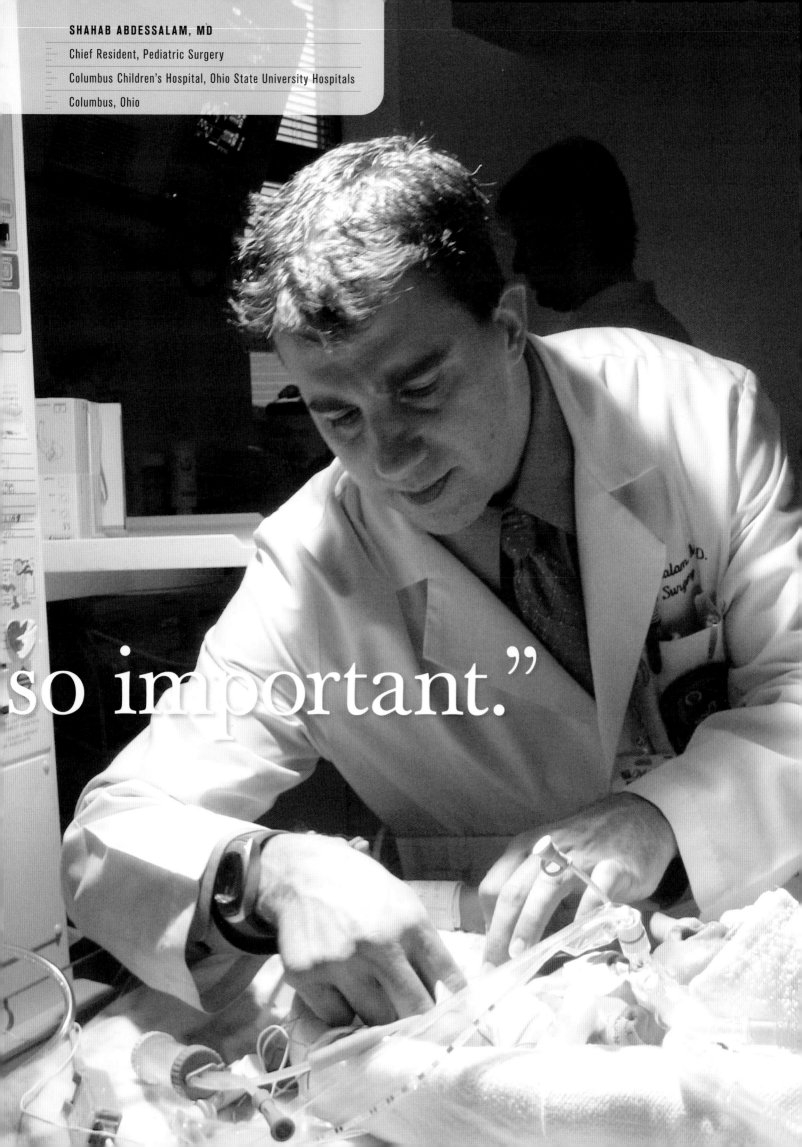

SHAHAB ABDESSALAM, MD

Chief Resident, Pediatric Surgery

Columbus Children's Hospital, Ohio State University Hospitals

Columbus, Ohio

so important."

the human body mixed with the complexities of cancer. So I thought surgical oncology would be what I wanted to do.

I went to the University of Nebraska Medical Center for general surgery and had every intention of going into surgical oncology. During my second year, I rotated through pediatric surgery and found that I just loved taking care of children. Children have no baggage. They come with an absolute innocence and purity, and I liked having an impact on that, and their recovery is unbelievable — they really bounce back well.

It is extremely difficult to get into pediatric surgery. There are a limited number of spots to match each year. For most of those positions, you have to spend two years in a basic science lab. By the time I had realized that I wanted to do pediatric surgery, it was too late for me to take two years off, and my residency program said no, we can't do that for you because of manpower. I was kind of bummed about that. So they said, well if you do surgical oncology that might be enough to get you into pediatric surgery. Surgical oncology was quite competitive as well. There were only 13 institutions that had surgical oncology spots. I was fortunate enough to match back at Ohio State. A year and a half was clinical, and then I spent a year and a half in a basic science lab. I got into a lab whose focus was tumor immunology, so it still dealt with cancer, but it also dealt with the immune system, which kind of fascinated me. The lab experience was extremely frustrating though, and I came to learn that basic science wasn't for me. It is full of multiple disappointments intermixed with infrequent success. My personality just couldn't handle repetitive failure. I do have a huge amount of respect, though, for those who are able to do that.

I was still interested in pediatric surgery, so now with my surgical oncology background and basic surgery, I was able to match my last year of surgical oncology, but the position for which I matched was a year and a half away, so I had another year to spend doing something. I had talked with Dr. Donna Caniano [program director of the pediatric surgery residency program at Ohio State University], and they had just started up a surgical critical care fellowship in pediatrics. So I said, well, that will do a couple of things. One, it gets me out of the lab and back to taking care of patients, which I love; two, it gets me back operating; and three, it gets me taking care of children, and taking care of the sickest ones would really sharpen up my skills overall. So I did that for a year and then continued here at Columbus Children's in pediatric surgery in July 2004.

As Dr. Caniano said, I've been a chief three times over: chief in general surgery, chief in surgical oncology, and chief in pediatric surgery. This is my 11th year since medical school.

Do you remember what your first day of your first residency was like?

I remember my first day [of general surgery] very well. My first rotation was in cardiothoracic surgery, and I remember being just scared out of my wits because now I was going to be taking care of very sick heart patients, and I really hadn't seen a patient in two months. I felt really, really green, but fortunately, I had a chief resident who was fantastic. The other good thing that happened was that two of the cardiothoracic surgeons had done their training at Ohio State. For some reason, they immediately liked me for that fact and kind of took me under their wing. I got to do so much on that service and learned so much. I was able to put sutures into a beating heart. As a brand new intern, I was on cloud nine, and it so much reaffirmed my going into surgery.

Role models are so critical. Whenever you have a bad rotation, nine times out of ten, it is coming from the top. That has always stuck with me. Now that I am in a senior position, I can have influence over what those underneath me are doing and how they are approaching the subject. I try to bring an element of humor so it is enjoyable and puts everybody at ease, and I try to get the best out of people and, I think, for the most part it is well received. The influences I had early on demonstrated that very well for me.

Were any moments from your first year of residency particularly memorable?

The fact that they tried to get me fired. Our residency program director hated me [chuckles] because I asked so many questions. I have had a lot of practice with this. When you ask questions of people who are unsure of themselves, they see it as an attack, and when they see it as an attack, they get extremely defensive. Medicine should not be that way. One of my attractions to medicine is that everything is not so clear cut. Nothing is ever black and white. I expect questions to be asked of me, and I expect the same of those around me. And if they can't defend what their actions are, then they shouldn't be doing it. Those who really don't feel good about their decisions see that as an attack and get very defensive. My residency director did not like my asking questions. He gave me a lot of grief that first year and made me keep quiet my whole second year.

When did you start feeling like a real doctor?

Oh, about three months ago [laughs]. Some would say I have stayed in training this long because I have never felt that confident. Residency offers one the opportunity of continued adolescence. There is always a "parent" overlooking your every move, and even nicer, someone you can turn to for advice. I don't think a majority of residency programs are long enough. I think a lot of physicians come out of their residencies and do a lot of on-the-job training, and that's scary for me as a surgeon. Any time you have to make a decision and act upon it, that's scary and I want to make sure I'm very good at it before I'm done. I've gone through peaks and plateaus and phases, where I think I can conquer the world, and then something comes along that humbles the hell out of me and puts me back in my place. I am so glad I am doing it under the guidance of someone else. And that is the beauty of residency: you can make a mistake or potentially make a mistake and have someone correct you. You have that protection. That's a beautiful thing. Someone told me in medical school that a surgeon by the name of [Robert Milton] Zollinger, one of the most famous surgeons that came out of Ohio State, said no one is trained until they have ten years of training. That always stuck with me.

What is it like being a chief resident?

The staff you are working with view you differently and tend to give you more respect. There is a fair bit more of administrative duties that you have to go through and learn, and that is important too, to be the boss and know how to work with a lot of different individuals. That is an art in itself, and it takes a while to learn that, too. When you have a bunch of eager med students and people looking to you for guidance, it is a good feeling.

How have you grown professionally and personally through your residency?

Oh boy, that is a tough question. I have definitely matured, no doubt. That is kind of a vague word, I know. I've definitely become a better listener. In between my second and third year I got married. My wife has given me a great deal of stability and is no doubt to whom I owe a majority of my success to. I have three children, ages six, four, and one. In the pediatric surgery world, that has allowed me to be a more compassionate physician because I can identify better than someone who doesn't have any children. My empathy level has gone way up as a result of that, and I am just a better person overall.

What has been the most meaningful part of your pediatric surgery residency?

Well, there are always individual cases that come to mind. The individual cases that have affected me the most are babies that come in who are extremely sick and have a problem, usually with their intestines, and need an operation, and you go in and fix the problem, and then, hopefully, you give the parents back a nice, healthy baby. I think the thing that has struck me the most is the understanding that the parents are going from a state of almost pure joy [after delivery] … then to have an ill baby … the emotional process for those parents is almost unimaginable. To have an impact on that, even if the outcome is not always good, and to be able make the process as manageable as possible has really brought meaning to my practice of medicine. Those are the toughest situations, I think, and something that has really, really hit home several times this year. Those are both some of the toughest, and also some of the most joyous cases. Just the relief and gratitude you can see on the parents' faces reaffirm my choice of profession.

Who has been most influential to you during your residency?

Well, I've really had a lot of influences. One of my biggest ones, starting back at medical school was one of the surgical oncologists, Dr. Edward Martin. He is the one who really latched onto me in medical school and got me passionate about surgical oncology. He was probably also very responsible for my matching at Ohio State in surgical oncology. When I approached him about going into pediatric surgery, he was just elated. I was kind of worried about how some of my mentors in surgical oncology would view my wanting to go into pediatric surgery, but he really understood and thought it was the greatest thing. He understood that children with cancer need specialized care just like adults with cancer. He saw the void in pediatric surgery as I did and knew that I could fill that void with my training in both surgical oncology and pediatric surgery. He helped me get this position as well. So he is definitely my most influential mentor and somebody I owe a lot of thanks to. He's a great physician — not only because he can operate on anything. The way he communicates with patients makes them feel like people, not patients, and his confidence as a surgeon lets residents make mistakes and allows them to fix those mistakes. Both of those attributes are great, and that is exactly the type of physician that I want to be.

Do you feel confident of your ability to practice independently once you finish your residency?

Yes, I do. I have a position back at the University of Nebraska at the Children's Hospital, an academic position. I will have residents working with me, which I knew I wanted in any job that I was looking at. I looked at several positions, and it really came down to one important thing. No matter what level of training you are at, whether it is medical school, residency, fellowship, or staff position, it is important to go to another location at each level. If you stay, you are always viewed at the level you were before. It is hard to break that mold, at least initially. In addition, the University of Nebraska was really where I fell in love in pediatric surgery. So I'm hoping to give that same influence to future generations of surgery residents. I will be working with residents at their early stages of development. If I can show them the beauty of surgical care of children, then I will have succeeded, as my mentors did for me.

What advice would you give new physicians who are starting their residencies?

Get the most out of your residency. Your residency isn't something you should take for granted or view as a job. You want to see as many patients as you can and as many disease processes, so your breadth of exposure is at its greatest. That way, when you see something unusual, you can say I saw that once before. If you've had that exposure, it is really helpful. I've obviously been a part of the transition to the 80-hour work week. One of the negative influences of this restriction is that I've seen too many residents more focused on going home and getting out of the hospital than on trying to get the most out of their residency, which can only be done by seeing lots of patients with lots of different diseases. Obviously there is a balance, but if you are the patient with the unusual disease, I think you would want a physician who has seen it all. Residency gives you that opportunity.

If you could change anything in medicine, what would that be?

People need to lighten up, no question about that. Medicine has to be an open forum. It has to be an area for discussion, and people cannot take offense to people's asking questions. Patients absolutely need to be able to ask questions, as well as your colleagues and residents and interns and medical students. If you don't understand something, you've got to be able to have a discussion about it. That is how you will get the best care for people. I think people are too afraid of hurting someone's feelings. It should be about getting at the best course of action.

Is there anything else you would like to add?

I have absolutely zero regrets about what I have done, and I would do it all over again. If I had to start medical school next week, I would do it again and take the same road again. As far as a chosen career, there is absolutely nothing better than pediatric surgery and having the additional training in surgical oncology makes taking care of children with cancer that much more satisfying. I can give them what I believe is the best possible care.

GIL BINENBAUM, MD

Chief Resident, Ophthalmology

Scheie Eye Institute, University of Pennsylvania

Philadelphia, Pennsylvania

"It's not about you,

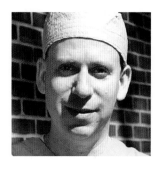

After six years as a Wall Street trader, Gil Binenbaum, MD, decided it was time for a change. He went back to school, completed his pre-med requirements and earned his medical degree at the University of Pennsylvania School of Medicine. He stayed there for his ophthalmology residency at the Scheie Eye Institute, where he served as chief resident in 2005–06. He also served as the resident member of the ACGME's Residency Review Committee for Ophthalmology.

Dr. Binenbaum is married with two children, Emi and Nate. His wife, Andrea, is a classical pianist and author. He enjoys spending time with his family and doing tai chi and meditation.

Why did you decide to change careers and go into medicine?

I was a foreign currency trader for six years on Wall Street in Manhattan. I basically wanted to go there to earn a fortune if I could, which is the only reason people go to Wall Street. I enjoyed it at first. It [foreign currency trading] was very high stress and fast-paced. I saw my materialistic motivation. With time, though, I started to realize it wasn't making me a happier person, and the basic bottom line is I decided to do something more meaningful with my life.

it's about the patient."

Years before, I had thought a bit about medicine when I started college. My father is a cardiologist, who was an engineer before that, and his mother, my grandmother, was a physician in Vienna in the early part of the twentieth century. About four years into my trading experience in Wall Street, I sort of had an epiphanistic experience. I was in a trading room. I had a phone board that had 200 buttons on it, and I could plug in on my phone and trade and be shouting numbers. In the midst of this, I suddenly had this clear picture of what had been pushing me on, and I recognized that the materialistic motivation in my life had lost its grip on me. Since then, for better or worse, money does not motivate me.

I enrolled in a post-grad pre-med program. I enrolled in Columbia University and started taking about one class a semester and working full-time. Soon I met up with a heart surgeon at Columbia, Mehmet Oz [author of *You: The Owner's Manual*]. Over the previous years, I had sort of developed a meditation practice — along with yoga and tai chi — for increasing your awareness. In retrospect, this practice really sort of led me towards the epiphany I had.

I became more interested in helping other people than in my own desires. That's the most honest description I can give you of my experience. Anyway, Mehmet offered to hire me as an assistant director of a research center to study using yoga, massage, hypnosis, etc., on people who were going to have cardiac surgery. I spent a year working for Mehmet; that's where I found my calling. I really felt that I could connect with people, and I felt great meaning with the seriousness of their conditions and the seriousness of the connections we could make.

I stopped working, which was really scary, went fulltime at Columbia, and ended up going back to Penn for medical school. I didn't really expect to go there. My wife and I had gotten an apartment in California so I could attend medical school there, and at the last minute I changed my mind. I was very impressed with the curriculum at Penn, which was very streamlined and systems-based. It appealed to me.

During medical school, at the end of first year we had a daughter, Emi. That was by far the most significant thing that happened to me. I started becoming involved in a number of curriculum committees because I had a sort of business/organizational background. I started thinking I might want to have an academic career.

What was the attraction of ophthalmology?

I was very confused. I liked a lot of different things about a lot of different fields, but I tried to think in a more global sense. I realized I really liked the operating room, and I liked outpatient clinics as well. I loved interacting with patients, especially children. I also liked solving problems in an immediate and longterm sense. I didn't quite as much care for inpatient management. Put that all together — that's what ophthalmology is.

"YOU NEED TO BE GIVEN THE OPPORTUNITY FOR INDEPENDENT DECISION-MAKING, BUT WITH GOOD SUPPORT."

What was the first day of your residency like?

Ophthalmology is a little different. We do a transitional year first. I did a few months of general surgery, a few months of general electives, and a month of ER. I was on call my very first day, and I was scared. In medical school, you don't really make all the decisions. You are really reviewing things with a resident. This was the first time I was called upon to make decisions on my own.

Parts of internship were exciting. I really liked my patient interactions, both because of my personality and because I was older. I felt being older affected my experience throughout medical school. I had already worked in the real world. I knew what it was like to go to a doctor as an adult non-physician. I had also already interacted with people in a work environment. Doctors don't always learn that as residents. I could definitely see a lot of fellow students and residents struggling with the realization that we are all working together, and just because someone has fewer years of school doesn't mean their job is any less important. I saw a lot of people with big egos doing that on Wall Street, and I still see people doing that in residency. In residency, you see, it's really about the patient, not about you.

It's very important when you are forced to be in a position to make a decision, right or wrong, to ask for assistance if you are really in over your head. You need to be given the opportunity for independent decision-making but with good support. You have to protect the patient, but you are going to make mistakes. You also need to make the mistakes. You won't learn about them unless you make them.

The first few months [of his ophthalmology residency] were much more difficult, much more daunting. Ophthalmology is a somewhat unique part of medicine. You simply don't learn much about the eye in medical school.

In ophthalmology, I remember Dr. Nicholas Volpe [the program director] giving us a little speech. He said that in the first few months of the residency, many people become discouraged and start to question or doubt why they went into this field. It really gets difficult. He said you just have to get over the hump. Once I got over the hump, I found ophthalmology everything I had hoped. You really have an impact on people's lives.

How is the chief year of your residency the same as and different from the first year of your ophthalmology residency?

I still feel like there are things I don't know, but I definitely know more than I did three years ago. I feel a lot more comfortable with the surgical aspects of ophthalmology. I think that the process over the course of the three years has been gradual. The demarcation between first and second and second and third isn't like a line in the sand. It's getting more subtleties of the surgery, more of the exam. It's not something you read in a book and you get it. I can look back and see how much more I know and see how little it is that [new first-year residents] know about ophthalmology. That is the most important thing to being an effective teacher, to see what it is that your students don't know. I feel like as a chief it is getting more difficult to put myself in the mindset of not knowing, but the effort is worthwhile.

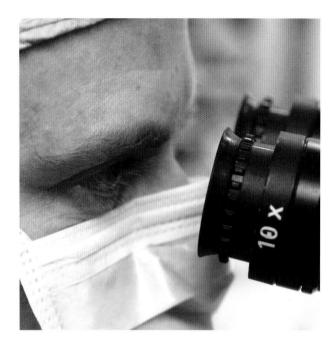
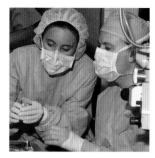
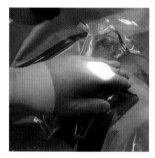

"YOU SHOULD TREAT EVERYONE YOU WORK WITH WITH THE SAME DEGREE OF RESPECT."

What advice would you give to medical students starting their residencies?

I would tell them that being scared doesn't mean you're incompetent. The most competent doctor is the one who has respect that things can go wrong. I don't honestly know if I am competent or not to practice by myself. I think I am, but I have to take for granted that the people who are training me and the accreditation body have done their jobs. They are supposed to prepare me to be on my own. And I can't know that because I am not on my own yet. I could be there, but I don't know.

It's very important to make decisions on your own, even if you're scared. You are going to make mistakes, and you need to make mistakes. You won't learn about them unless you make them. The corollary to that is to know when to ask for help. Don't be stubborn or embarrassed. It's not about you, it's about the patient. It's important to be given the opportunity for independent decision-making but with good backup support. It's very important when you are forced to be in a position to make a decision, right or wrong, to ask for assistance if you are really in over your head.

Another point I would make is you should treat everyone you work with with the same degree of respect. People should try to remember the altruistic reason they went into medicine and take the compassionate approach to anyone they are dealing with and to remember the most irritating or demanding patient is the one who is probably the most scared, and not to take it personally.

Have any moments been particularly meaningful in your chief residency year?

The first time I could go through a cataract surgery case completely by myself, I felt a sense of achievement. If you can't do the whole surgery, you can't practice independently where you can't have someone bail you out. It really was a big deal.

Along the same lines, being able to interact with the patients and seeing the degree of thankfulness and gratitude and praise for basically restoring their sight … I found it very humbling, and it reaffirmed the reason I went into medicine in the first place.

Being on the Residency Review Committee for Ophthalmology during the residency has been very rewarding as well. It is a committee where there is a real tangible effect to your decision. It impacts not just on a resident's experience but also on the program directors and faculty. I very much enjoy the opportunity to be involved in that. The people on the RRC have treated me as a colleague, and not as a student.

If you could change one thing in medicine, what would you change?

I would do away with all the health insurance companies and would create a national health plan so that every single person had insurance. The health plan would be financed by the government, and every single health decision would be made by a physician. There would be no issues of coverage or no coverage. I understand there are limited resources, but it would be the doctors' decision on how those resources are allocated.

Is there anything else you would like to say?

I am doing a fellowship in pediatric ophthalmology and strabismus at the Children's Hospital of Philadelphia. I hope ultimately to base my practice in a pediatric hospital, working with patients and training students, residents, and fellows. I like being in a setting where I'm interacting with people who aren't in ophthalmology and being on the cutting edge of things. I also would like to be involved in organized ophthalmology and medical education in some way to improve the way that people learn ophthalmology.

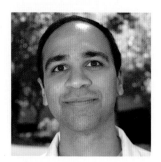

V ishal Gala, MD, credits his grandfather for sparking his interest in medicine. He remembers visiting his grandfather, a physician, in Mumbai, India, and observing the compassionate way he cared for his patients. Dr. Gala was born in Buffalo, New York, but has spent most of his life in Michigan. He earned a bachelor's degree from the University of Michigan, majoring in economics and biology, and then went on to medical school at the University of Michigan, where he graduated as class valedictorian. Dr. Gala was the resident representative to the ACGME's Residency Review Committee for Neurosurgery and chair of the ACGME's Committee of Review Committee Residents. Following the completion of his residency, Dr. Gala began a fellowship in minimally invasive spine surgery at the University of Chicago Hospitals.

How did you become interested in medicine and what drew you to neurosurgery?

My parents are originally from India, and my grandfather was a family practitioner in India and had a clinic that was attached to the apartment that my grandparents lived in. I have traveled to India probably every other year since I was a child, and so for years I watched my grandfather work as a family physician, and he was really very much the old fashioned family "doc." He would make house calls, he would see people at all hours of the day and night. What I noticed most was the respect he received from everyone in the community and the sort of the standing he had within the community, and I was always in awe of that. I used to see what he did and how he would help people who were sick. At a young age, it really made an impression on me.

"Maintaining perspective is

So I always thought about becoming a doctor, and I would say that was really my original inspiration for going into medicine. As I went through high school and college I really developed an interest in the sciences and felt that medicine would be the best for me because I thought it would provide me with the personal satisfaction of helping others and provide a social good, but also satisfy my interest in science and my intellectual curiosity.

When I got to college, I started doing research. I worked in a surgical lab where I did a lot of animal surgery, and that is when I became really interested in surgery. When I started medical school I was pretty intent on becoming some kind of surgeon. I was not really sure what kind, and then during my medical school I really became interested in neurosciences and

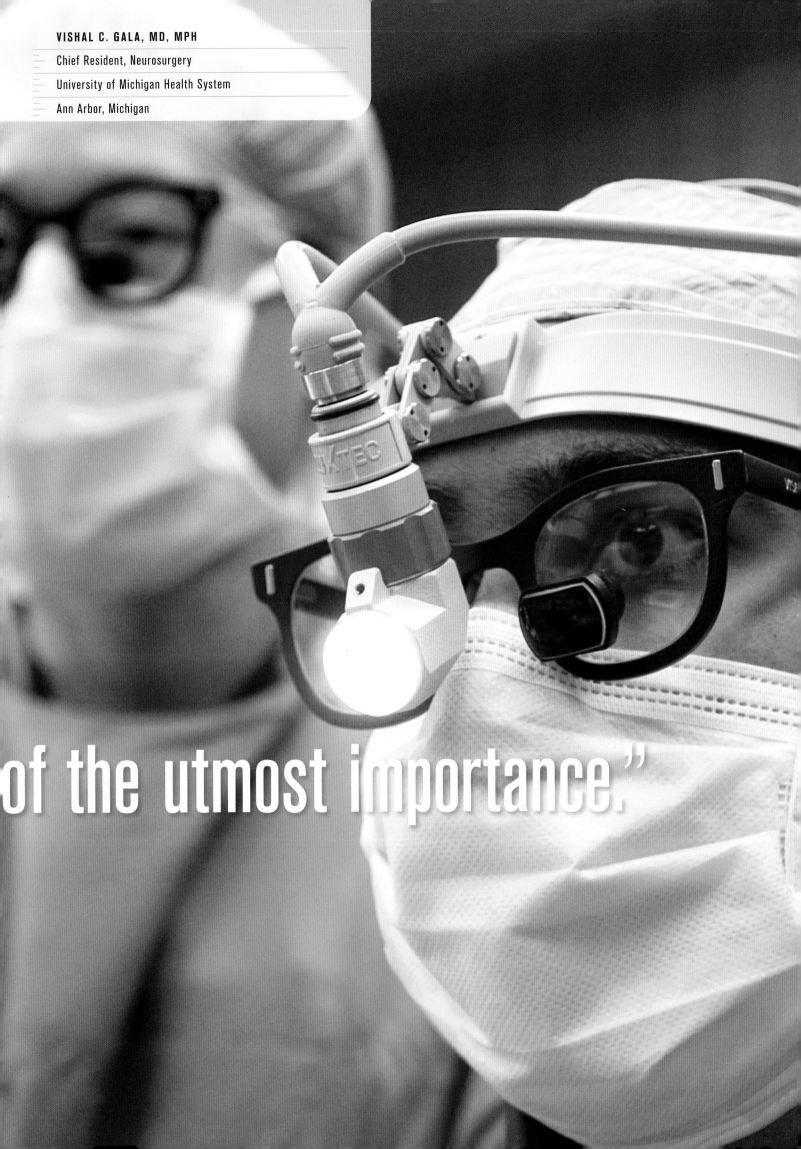

VISHAL C. GALA, MD, MPH

Chief Resident, Neurosurgery

University of Michigan Health System

Ann Arbor, Michigan

of the utmost importance."

decided to do neurosurgery as an elective in my third year, and that is really when I fell in love with it. I felt it was a great combination of the cognitive aspects of medicine and being a good neurologist but also being a surgeon and being able to have an objective and being able to achieve it with an operation. I also felt like neurosurgery was kind of one of the true frontier fields of medicine. I mean, neurosurgery is probably one of the youngest specialties in all of medicine, and there is still so much to be learned about the nervous system and so many applications of new technology that we use in neurosurgery, with image guidance in cranial surgery and new instrumentation and techniques in the spine.

I have done all my training at the University of Michigan. I did college, medical school and my residency here. I am chief resident; this is my seventh year of training. I did a one-year general surgery internship followed by a six-year neurosurgery residency, which included 18 months of research time, which is when I did my master's degree in public health.

What was the first year of your residency like?

You come out of medical school after a fairly relaxed fourth year and then all of a sudden you are an intern: you are wearing a long coat, you have an MD next to your name, and all of a sudden nurses and everybody who partially ignored you for months [laughs] are now asking you real questions, and people are actually going to obey your orders and institute them. It was a little daunting at first.

When I first started, I was certainly nervous, I think, as everyone is when they start their residency, as to whether they are truly prepared to be real doctors and actually have the final say. The thing I remember the most is that the nurse or somebody would ask you a question and it was your call, you were going to give the order and it was going to be instituted and somebody was going to get a medication based on your decision. Understanding that responsibility was the most nerve-wracking thing of starting.

It is interesting: over the year, at some point, especially because you work so hard as an intern and spend so much time at the hospital — especially back in the pre-80-hour era, which I am a part of — the internship was a pretty intense experience and you came up to speed relatively quickly. I remember that I was told by one of our surgery professors that at some point during the year — you will not know when it happens — all of a sudden you will be pretty comfortable taking care of pretty sick people, at least keeping them going through the night and taking care of basic problems. And it is true. It happens. There was a point where all of a sudden I became much more confident and comfortable, at least with the basics of taking care of very sick people in the hospital and the ICU, preoperatively, postoperatively. It was a real great experience.

What do you remember from the first year of your neurosurgery residency?

Neurosurgery is a bit of an island. There is not a lot of overlap that you learn when you are doing your general surgery internship about how we do things in neurosurgery. I mean, certainly there are the basics of pre- and postoperative care, but the operations we perform are obviously very different. The tools we use are totally different, the way we manage patients for the particular conditions they have is often very different than in general surgery. I only did about six weeks of neurosurgery during my internship, so, aside from what I had done as a medical student, it was all very new to me. It was pretty daunting. In neurosurgery we rely heavily on interpreting our own imaging studies, so I had to learn very quickly how to read CT scans, how to read MRI scans, how to interpret them on my own. When I am on call I make decisions based on those scans and my assessment of a patient's neurologic exam. So again, it was a real growing process, and I think the learning curve my first year of neurosurgery was very steep. I did a fair number of basic operations, learning how to do the real basics of what you do in neurosurgery, particularly on call at night, when people have life-threatening neurologic conditions — evaluating trauma, and things like that. So it was a real steep learning curve for me that first year, but after that first year of neurosurgery, I felt at least somewhat confident that I could deal with most things in neurosurgery that we see on call at night.

Did you feel confident that you would learn all that you needed to know to become a competent neurosurgeon?

Yes. Neurosurgery is a long residency. It is seven years long and with good reason. There really is a lot to learn in neurosurgery: we cover the brain, the spine, the peripheral nerves, and it really is a lot in seven years. It is a real system of graduated responsibility. I knew that I had a lot to learn, but by seeing how my colleagues and the older residents were doing and progressing through the program, I felt fairly confident that over the seven years I would learn everything that I needed to. Now that I am chief, I have to say that is absolutely true. I have had a great experience; it has been a real system of graduated responsibility, both in terms of operating and patient care responsibilities, and I do feel that by the end of this year I will be competent to practice independently. Absolutely.

How is your chief residency year different from and the same as the previous years of your residency?

Well, as the chief resident, especially in neurosurgery programs, which tend to be very small, the chief residents have a huge role in running the day-to-day activities of the service. The chief resident has a primary responsibility for all the patients that are in the hospital. The chief resident conducts rounds, along with the junior residents, every morning and every afternoon and directs the care of all the patients on the service. Also, the chief resident has the administrative responsibilities to delegate tasks to the appropriate resident or intern, also to assign cases in the operating room each day, cover our in-patient clinics, as well as consultations in the emergency department. The chief resident typically does the most complex cases each day that are performed. And so, as a chief resident, you really are given the opportunity to have more independence, more responsibility, really to take charge and to provide care for the patients — under the supervision, still, of the staff, but largely under your own control. I certainly think the staff also relies heavily on the chief resident to provide that care, given that they are all very busy with all these different activities and responsibilities that they have. The service and the staff really rely on the chief resident to essentially run the show.

Is there any particular moment that stands out in your chief resident year?

I think what has impressed me most this year is the amount of autonomy I now have in the operating room. I spend more time operating independently; I am given more autonomy to start cases and do cases on my own — of course still under supervision, but doing much more of the case on my own. Also, I am taking junior residents through cases and teaching junior residents how to do some basic cases in neurosurgery and actually feeling comfortable doing that. The most striking thing to me this year is the improvement in my surgical skills and the fact that I feel confident doing a wide variety of procedures, largely on my own.

How do you feel you have grown, both personally and as a doctor, during your residency?

As a doctor, it is pretty clear. My knowledge of medicine and particularly of neurosurgery has steadily grown over the seven years, and I feel like each year I have gotten better and better, and I really feel like my chief year has really been the culmination of that seven-year experience.

As a person, I have grown a great deal as well. Seven years is a long time. You go from your mid-twenties to your early thirties [laughs]. You know, in neurosurgery, we do deal with a lot of difficult conditions: people who have life-threatening illnesses. We unfortunately deal with a lot of people who have catastrophic conditions, trauma or hemorrhages, a lot of end-of-life issues. From a personal standpoint, my ability to talk to people, to patients and their families, has really improved over seven years, and that is by virtue by being in training and having to provide care for patients that are this sick and having the responsibility as a resident, particularly as the chief resident, to be the primary contact between patients and families. I think I have become much better at handling these types of difficult situations. I also think that the chief year has sort of thrust me into more of a leadership position, and I think the whole experience together, combined with the chief year, has really made me more confident and a better leader and a better administrator and a better doctor.

Who was influential to you during your residency?

It is hard for me to pinpoint one specific person. I think I have probably taken away something from each and every member of our faculty. You know, as far as residencies go, neurosurgery departments tend to be small. We have had about 10 to 12 faculty here during my whole residency, and over seven years you get to know people fairly well. We only work with each other and 12 other residents during our residencies. I would say, having worked closely with these 10 or 12 people, that I really learned something from each and every one of them, and that ranges from medical care to surgical technique to basic management to how to deal with patients and families. I find myself, particularly in my chief year now when I am thrust in these situations, whether it is in the operating room or in the intensive care unit or whether it is during a family discussion, utilizing pearls that I have gleaned from each of these people in different situations.

The one person that has been very supportive of my career has been my chairman, Dr. Hoff, who has been the chairman here for many years and was a real role model for me when I was in medical school and interested in going into neurosurgery. He is the one who supported

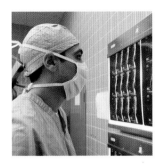
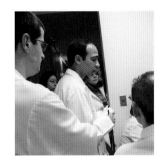
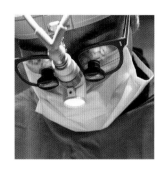

"THERE IS STILL SO MUCH TO BE LEARNED ABOUT THE NERVOUS SYSTEM."

my nomination to the RRC for Neurosurgery, which led me to go on and become involved with the resident council and the ACGME, and he has really supported my development in organized medicine and residency education.

What advice would you give to medical school graduates starting their residencies?

I think it is very easy over a seven-year period of time to become jaded and to lose your humanity a little bit. Residency can be a very intense experience; it can be overwhelming. You are inundated with work every single day, and many times in many fields you are dealing with a lot of sick patients. I think you start, to some degree, to see all the patients as work and as obstacles to your being able to go home and carry on with your life, and I think it is important to recognize that and to understand these are real people: this is somebody's mom, somebody's sister, somebody's brother, somebody's child. Maintaining that perspective is really of the utmost importance. Those who become jaded no longer enjoy medicine and forget why they went into medicine. So I think that maintaining that sense of humanity and compassion is really the most important thing through the course of your residency.

If there was one thing you could change in medicine, what would that be?

The one thing that is most striking to me, particularly having seen the practice of medicine in India with my grandfather and comparing how the practice of medicine is there to the practice of medicine here, is that the litigious nature of our society really undermines in many ways the basic patient-doctor relationship here. Because of the great fear of litigation and malpractice, defensive medicine is practiced universally throughout the country. It results in spending excess resources where we probably do not need to just because we are practicing defensive medicine. It has resulted in real barriers to care for many people, where physicians opt not to practice or provide certain services in certain states and communities due to fear of litigation and being unable to acquire malpractice insurance. Always having that concern in the back of your mind, I think, is the one thing that sometimes sours that doctor-patient relationship and makes it not quite the same. It is not the vision people had of what practicing medicine would be like when they started. It is hard no to be a little cynical by the time you are done.

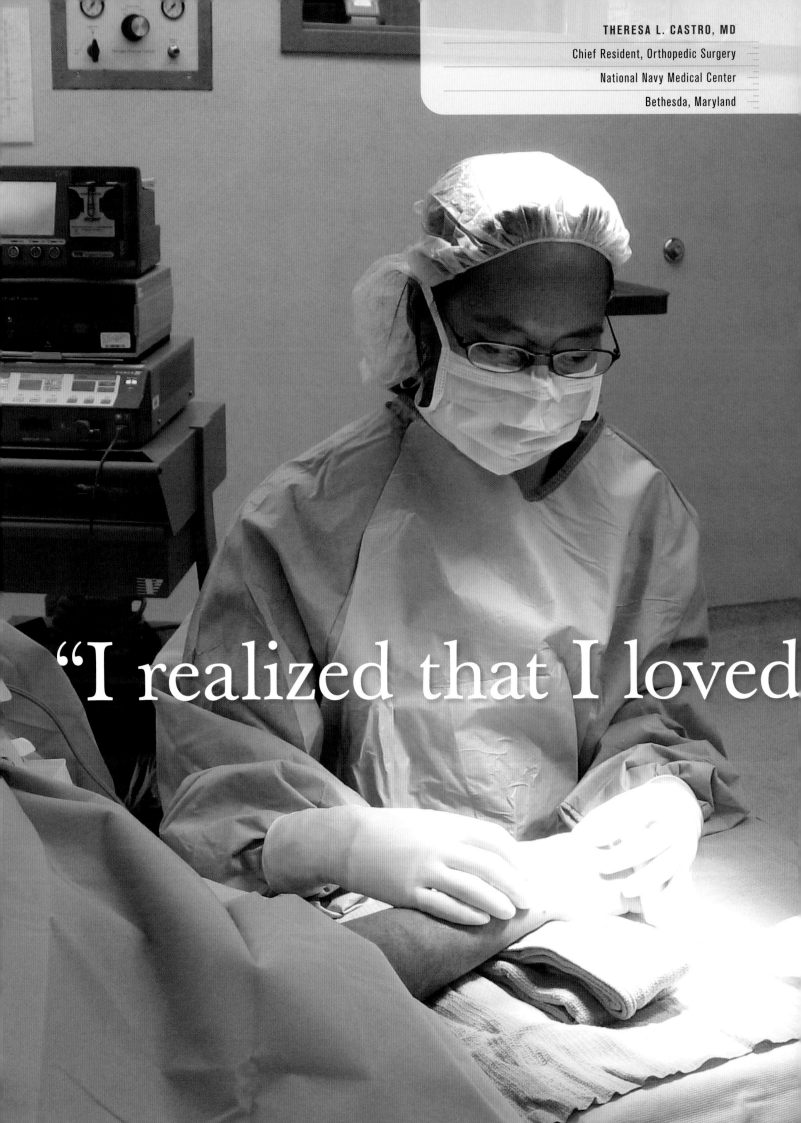

THERESA L. CASTRO, MD

Chief Resident, Orthopedic Surgery

National Navy Medical Center

Bethesda, Maryland

"I realized that I loved

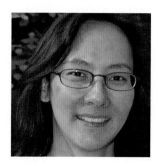

W hen Theresa Castro, MD, was a biochemistry major at the University of California at Davis, she realized that medicine included all the things that she was looking for in a career. The daughter of a retired Navy chief — she was born in Inchon, Korea — Dr. Castro decided to join the Navy. In March 2003, when the United States invaded Iraq, she was in her first year of her orthopedic surgery residency at the National Navy Medical Center. Caring for the influx of wounded soldiers and sailors changed her residency and her outlook on life.

Following graduation, Dr. Castro was assigned to the United States Navy Base at Guantanamo Bay, Cuba. In her free time, Dr. Castro enjoys hiking and biking.

Why did you decide to become a physician?

I was not one of those little kids who always grew up thinking I want to be a doctor. It was something I came across in college because I definitely liked the sciences, and I thought, It was really neat to work in a hospital and help people. I can't imagine doing anything else than being a doctor. This is the perfect field that kind of combines the sciences and doing actual hands-on stuff and seeing people. It just appeals to me for those reasons.

the operating room."

I worked as a chemist for seven years. Then I applied to medical school and got into the military medical school, and a civilian one as well, and just for financial purposes, decided to go the military route. My dad's a retired Navy chief and my brother was in the military at the time, so it seemed like a fairly normal thing to do.

In the Navy, it's a little different. Your residency is broken up, so you do an internship a year after you graduate from medical school and then go out to the fleet or some unit and serve as a GMO, a general medical officer, and essentially you're a family practice doc or a general practitioner for a bunch of sailors or soldiers. So after I did my one year of internship, I went out with the Seabees, which is the construction battalion that builds for the Navy, and went to Okinawa for two deployments. I reapplied for residency while serving, and then I got into the orthopedic residency here.

Photographs: left, courtesy of the U.S. Navy; right, Michael Frew

What drew you to orthopedic surgery?

In medical school the first few years are mostly classroom and the last two are clerkships. When I started doing my clerkship, I realized that I loved the operating room and I did not particularly like clinic, per se. In other words, internal medicine was definitely not something that appealed to me. I liked operating. At our medical school, you get two weeks of orthopedics as a surgical sub-clerkship during your third year of medical school. During mine, half the attendings were at the academy meeting or away, so I just really didn't get a great exposure to it. I thought that it's kind of a male field; it's for guys who like building things, and I don't build things. I just didn't think it was something that I would be proficient in.

I actually was planning to do general surgery all through the end of medical school, and even through most of my internship. As a general surgery intern, you have to rotate through orthopedics for a month. As luck would have it, a lot of the residents were out of town at a conference. I got to scrub for a lot of cases and got some face time with the attendings and some of the senior residents and thought this is what I want to do. It's concrete. It's broken people; you fix them. Most of the patients are pretty healthy, so it appealed to me. It didn't have the acute situations that general surgeons have to deal with, managing sick patients, because that's not what I wanted to do. I love the surgery. There's soft tissues; it's not all bone, and there's a lot of subspecialties within orthopedics.

In the military, we don't do the match, so basically you're kind of forced to apply to all the orthopedic programs within the Navy, and I chose Bethesda because that's where I had the most exposure, knew the most people.

What did you feel like on the first day of your orthopedic residency?

It was very exciting. It's funny because I remember coming here and meeting one of my counterparts — there's three of us in my class. And I met George, one of my two counterparts, for the first time when we were checking in. We sat and had lunch, and we were so happy to be here, because it is competitive. There are a lot of other factors that they take into account: prior service and other, less tangible things. It was extremely exciting and very frightening. I felt absolutely terrified to get my first consult in the emergency room for a fractured wrist. I just did not feel like I was in my element, but I knew I wanted to be here.

Everything was just going swimmingly until Operation: Iraqi Freedom started. The tone and the content of our residency changed forever. This residency has always been renowned in the Navy as being kind of the ivory tower. Our groups tend to score very high, we've never had failures, even though we're not a level one trauma center. They have to send us out for that. It was kind of a relaxed atmosphere, and then all of a sudden this war started and we went from having maybe five or ten patients on the ward to 45 patients on the ward with multiple extremity traumas requiring multiple washouts and debridements of amputations that had gone bad.

It was a rude awakening. I would be rounding on patients and taking down their dressings for the first time at 10 p.m. I saw open fractures, segmental losses, parts of hands, feet, *many* amputations, many above the knees, many below the knee. And of course, these people all had head injuries and other things, so a lot of them were in the ICU. In normal trauma hospitals, orthopedics usually isn't the admitting service for these, but maybe 80–90 percent of these patients had orthopedic injuries with concomitant belly issues or other injuries. We ended up admitting them on our service and managing them. We had general surgery consulting, but we were essentially the primary service for a lot of these. It was a big wakeup call for this hospital, because the status quo was "we" — as in, whoever is working here — want to get out at a decent hour, and we don't want to do cases at night. There were times when we had multiple operating rooms with junior residents in there working on some of our wounded Marines. That was hard.

When Operation: Iraqi Freedom II happened the following year and a half, and we got the new wave, it was a different story, because our hospital by that time had learned to come up with a system. It changed this hospital and it changed this residency.

How did the experience change you?

It changed my experience for the good. Somehow I think we were lucky enough to still come out and still get a good, well-rounded education orthopedically, as far as the elective-type procedures. We still had a total joint rotation, we were still seeing hand patients, and they sent us away for peds. So our group still ended up getting a good education.

"THE TONE AND THE CONTENT OF OUR RESIDENCY CHANGED FOREVER."

I think from a deeper perspective I certainly feel for these patients, and I felt like everything that I did was important. Not that it wasn't before, but these are people whose lives are forever changed. You know this is someone who's not going to walk again or whose arm is blown off. This is stuff we hadn't seen before. People who were dying before from head injuries or visceral injuries are living, but they're coming back with three and four extremity injuries. And they're bad ones, too. They're just — it was just [sighs] — in one extremity you'd have like 20 holes with shrapnel and broken bones and the nerve is out here, and it's not just the nerve that needs to be re-approximated, there's an 8-centimeter segmental loss.

Infection is a big thing. *Acinetobacter* is a gram-negative bacteria that's found in almost all these injured in the Middle East, in Afghanistan as well as Iraq. Many of their wounds become infected and, if not, they're definitely colonized.

Usually, by the time they get to us, they're probably going to live. This is not a place where many of them died, because by the time they made it us they had gone from the field to one of four surgical places, then to Germany, and then they were flown here. So it was more like how are we going to keep these people clear of infection, get them healthy and then get their wound closed. You know, if we can get their wounds closed and healed and not infected, then one to six months down the road we can deal with their tendon transfers or their nerve repairs. Because the war's been going on for a few years we're seeing these patients back with us. I see patients that I remember from two years ago who are coming back and getting osteotomies or tendon transfers for injuries that they incurred in 2004.

I realized that it made me less selfish, and I think made me more acutely aware that there are bigger things than my own comfort and optimal learning experience. You have to take what's given to you and get through it because no matter how hard it is for us or how late we're up, these people have it a lot harder. And I feel like my two counterparts, George and Brion, felt the same way. We're happy — I don't know if "happy" is the word — but I think we feel proud or grateful that we are part of this and that we can help. They keep trickling in, so it's also depressing. You feel sorry for them.

When you started your residency, did you feel confident that you would learn everything you needed to learn to become an orthopedic surgeon in independent practice?

If we'd had this conversation last year, I'd say absolutely not, I didn't get enough hand surgery [laughs]. But our hand rotation is during our chief year, and I'm doing that right now, and I'm getting a ton of hand surgery. It is a great rotation. We've changed it so now our juniors go through this rotation earlier. I had good peds, I had great trauma, and by trauma I mean true, real trauma, community trauma. We have Shock Trauma at Baltimore for four months, and we also go to Washington Hospital Center. There's nothing that really scares me anymore because this war started before I went to Shock Trauma and when I went there, there was nothing this bad. There just wasn't! Improvised explosive devices mess people up badly; it's worse than a motorcycle and it's worse than a car accident.

The other thing I've learned is that nobody has all the answers. There are problems that I don't think anyone knows the right answer for. I think the answer is talking to your peers, talking to people who know more than you and getting their opinions. These are not standard injuries where someone says, "Well, of course you must do this." These are injuries that people just typically haven't seen before, where a whole large part of the femur is gone, the hip is gone. You learn by experience and by talking to people. That's why I think the Internet's great because you can email X-rays and you can talk to people you've networked with. Some of our local civilian ortho-trauma guys have pitched in and helped us too, which was great.

After I graduate I'm going out to Guantanamo Bay, Cuba, for a year to be the only orthopedic surgeon there. I'll see the detainees and the people who are stationed there, as well as civilian contractors. I'm the only ortho there, so it's kind of daunting. I think I'll be okay. I know that a phone call away or an e-mail picture away are all my contacts here, and there are two great hand surgeons here. There are people I've met other places that I can bounce this stuff off of. That's part of surgery: you never stop learning, you don't get to a point of, "Yeah, now I know everything."

What is it like being a chief resident?

Our program is so small, there are only three of us, so there is no chief resident, it's just our chief resident year. Each of us takes four months where we are the administrative chief. But we're all equal.

On my typical day, we meet up on the wards at about six in the morning, and we make rounds. Then we go down for a morning conference. That's usually an academic conference, and we start out with the junior residents presenting anything that came in the night before to let us know what's going on so they can be critiqued. After that we break and then we go to the operating room if it's our OR day or we go to the clinic if it's a clinic day. There's always a washout, so if the chief who's doing the ortho-trauma is on vacation or gone, we just kind of fill in for each other. The gist is to get the work done. I actually usually leave, on average, by 5 p.m. or 5:30 p.m. My life this year is wonderful now. The first four months were not so wonderful because I was the ortho-trauma chief, and I did all the Operation Iraqi Freedom patients. It kind of picked up in the summer — we started getting more casualties — and it was crazy.

Now it is a wonderful time. In addition to the three of us, there's one from the year below us sharing chief call, so I'm only on call, on average, every four nights. Now that it's slowed down in terms of the wounded coming in, most of the time I don't have to come in during the middle of the night. It's a big difference from junior year. Junior year, you're here all the time, and you're trying not to get yelled at [laughs] and trying to do all the scut work and make sure you have films.

I have more autonomy now. I have more time to read. More time to spend with my friends and family, which is important too.

Has there been anything about your chief residency year that has been particularly meaningful?

You walk into your chief residency year and suddenly people trust you to do cases. I myself am a little shocked, like what happened between one day and the other? I'm sure it didn't happen like that, but it just seems that way. It's kind of exciting, and I guess that has made a big impression on me.

The thought processes go from beginning as a junior: I'm doing things because I don't want to get in trouble to [as a chief resident] I'm doing things because I want to do the case right.

Has there been anyone who has been particularly influential to you throughout your residency?

As far as an attending, it's Francis McGuigin, one of our staff who's getting ready to retire. He's our foot and ankle surgeon, though he actually does a lot of general orthopedic surgery, a lot of trauma. About a month into our residency we had a retreat. He gave a talk about what a privilege it is to be here. He said our ultimate responsibility is the patient, and to learn. He said you have to read an article every night. This is the person who's taught me, as painful as it's been, off and on, to be a good surgeon and to do right by the patient. You can see it with his dealings with the patients. He is the kind of surgeon I want to be. He is one that says "Go the extra step, stay the extra hour, talk to the patient, do what you have to do, make sure everything is right." Don't foul up so the patient is lying there under general anesthesia for an hour because you didn't make sure the equipment was there.

I also have a sort of life mentor, two really, Patricia and Dan Solin. Patricia grew up in my hometown, family friends, she babysat me. She's about 15 years older, a successful upper manager at some firm at the time. My mom would constantly hold her up to my sister and me as the example of what we could achieve if we went to college. Her husband, Dan, has been above and beyond supportive. When I felt like I had been working as a chemist for too long and was thinking that I didn't want to take the MCAT, didn't know if I wanted to go to medical school, didn't know if I was smart enough, Dan said that I absolutely must do it. They've been my strongest advocates through every step of the way. They came to my residency graduation last month.

"THE OTHER THING I'VE LEARNED IS THAT NOBODY HAS ALL THE ANSWERS."

What advice would you give to medical school graduates who are starting their residencies?

Just to be honest and don't lie. That sounds ridiculous because we like to think of doctors as generally being honest people. But it's a stressful field, and it's very competitive and there are a lot of people asking "Did you do this? Did you listen to the heart? Did you check this?" You want to say yes, so one of the things I learned early on is you've just got to be honest. Once people know you can't be believed, then people aren't going to trust you. You owe it to your patients to tell the truth and to report what you saw, and if you didn't do something, it's okay to say you didn't. There's such a temptation to just tell people what they want to hear because you're answering to so many people.

The other thing is, if there's something bothering you when you're ready to turn off that light, this little, Hey, I should check it, you have just got to do it because no one else is going to do it. Work hard, go the extra mile. If you were supposed to follow up on something but you have to clock out because of the 80-hour work week rule, make sure you talk to somebody that is going to be there. Make a good turnover.

The third component is thinking of every patient as your grandmother. This sounds so stupid, but it's so true. You're tired, you've operated all day. You don't want to go talk to family members who are going to ask you 300 questions. As residents, we like to say, "Well, that's the attending's job!" Well, sometimes attendings forget to do it or they just don't. I tell myself that I had the privilege of cutting in that person's body. At the very least, I can go talk to the family. People can learn techniques and get technically better, but you can't learn to be a decent person.

What is one thing that could be changed or improved in medicine? What is one thing you think medicine does particularly well?

Oh, goodness. It's hard to speak for that, because I think I'm somewhat protected being in the military. If we want to order something and we think that it's appropriate, nobody says no, at least not at this hospital. So I can speak from the military medicine aspect. It's a good system, not perfect by any means. There's no financial incentive, so I think this allows us to be better at indicating elective surgeries, which translates as better care for the patients.

Do you plan to have a career in the military?

I do. I owed them seven years for the four years of free medical school. I paid back two of those as a general medical officer, so now I owe them five more.

I like being in the military. I don't think I ever thought I would say this, but I think it's changed me. It's given me an appreciation for our duty. If you ask people in the military who are physicians, they will say that they're physicians first and foremost. But the reality is that we're commissioned military officers who are there to make sure the mission gets done. Somehow we have to find a way to reconcile our jobs as doctors with our jobs as military officers. It's tricky. I think I have a greater appreciation for that sometimes-difficult pathway and trying to walk that fine line between doing the right thing and respecting the privacy of the patients and doing what I think I should do as a doctor for patients and also, at the same time, recognizing and supporting the mission of the unit.

I am appreciative of the military and the Navy. They have given me great experiences and a great education.

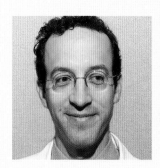

A high school anatomy course hooked Bryan Voelzke, MD, on a medical career, and the opportunity to do both surgery and clinical work and develop longterm relations with patients drew him to urology. The Texas native earned a bachelor's degree in biology from Baylor University and his medical degree from the University of Texas Health Science Center in San Antonio. He began his urology residency at Loyola University Medical Center in Maywood, Illinois in 2000 and served as chief resident of urology in 2005–06. Dr. Voelzke will complete a one-year fellowship in Melbourne, Australia and then enter a trauma and male reconstructive fellowship at the University of California-San Francisco in 2007.

In his free time, Dr. Voelzke enjoys biking, golfing and fly fishing.

"I LIKE THAT YOU ARE

Why did you decide to go into medicine?

No one in my family has gone into medicine. No one was pushing me to go into it. My parents were pretty indifferent as long as I went to college. I grew up always enjoying science. There was an anatomy course we could take our senior year in high school. I loved the anatomy course, and the physiology of how things worked caught my attention. By the start of my freshman year in college, I knew that medicine was for me. Since then I have become more enamored with medicine since it is such a dynamic and constantly changing field. If you don't keep up, you are left behind. I also enjoy getting to know people and establishing a kind of rapport with them.

I worked as an operating room technician in college during the summers, which essentially amounted to my retracting organs during surgical procedures. My favorite job was to hold the heart still while the surgeons sutured in their anastomoses for heart bypass surgery. With surgery, I liked that you got to work with your hands, fix things, and make an immediate impact on someone else. In some surgical fields, you operate and send them back to their cardiologist or primary care provider, but I found that in urology you will essentially follow most of your patients for life after operating on them. I have found that most surgical fields have an associated quirk that people associate with surgeons within the field. With urology, it is hard to be arrogant about specializing in the urinary system. Most people who go into urology tend to be relaxed and laid back, and I liked that when doing my surgical clerkships in medical school.

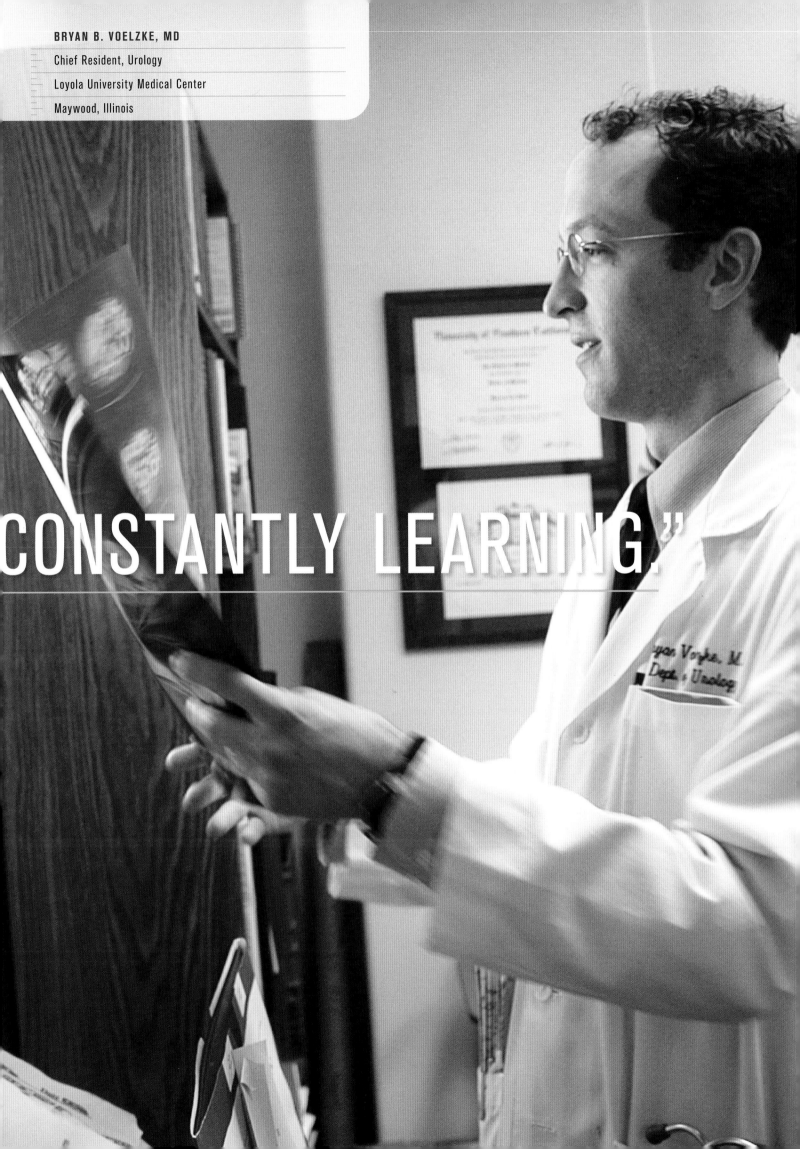

BRYAN B. VOELZKE, MD

Chief Resident, Urology

Loyola University Medical Center

Maywood, Illinois

CONSTANTLY LEARNING."

Loyola was my top choice [for residency]. I had always lived in Texas. I'm not married so I pretty much had my choice where I could go, and I figured it would be a nice thing to experience another state. People told me that you would interview and have an instinct that you would fit in at certain programs. I got that feeling when I went to Loyola, and luckily they accepted me for a residency position in 2000.

I've been very happy my last six years. I enjoy Chicago; it's a great town. Dr. Flanigan, our chairman, has a great way of working with the residents. He values our opinions. There definitely is a feeling that you can talk to the attendings in our program, that your information is valued. There's not a big chasm between the residents and the attendings where you are made to feel like an inferior human being. That has made coming to work an enjoyable experience even when the hours are long and tiring.

What was the first day of your residency like?

I started out in the surgical ICU. It was very overwhelming. The first order I signed was a death certificate. I guess someone had expired the night before, and it wasn't at all what I was expecting. It was very fast-paced. The number of patients we had to cover was very large; there were three intensive care units. The shifts were 24 hours on, 24 hours off, but if felt more like 36 hours on and 12 hours off. I would be gone the next day, and everything would change. There would be new trauma patients, and it was like having to relearn everything all over each day. I was amazed that the upper-level residents could come in and absorb the information and know what to do. I realized, looking back, that you have to establish the framework of what is important and what is not. When you're an intern, you're trying to remember every piece of information. It was one of the more challenging rotations to start off with. I didn't know it at the time.

When did you start feeling like a doctor?

It was just a gradual process — not any defining moment. By the end of my intern year, I felt like I was a doctor who was more clinically adept. As a chief resident, I am still learning. I fully expect it will remain that way after I graduate. I don't ever want to take the philosophy that I know everything; that is the biggest mistake you can make.

Does any moment stand out from the first year of your residency?

I was three months into my residency and on the cardiovascular service at our affiliated veterans' hospital. I was walking up to the surgical ICU, and I noticed a patient that our fellow had performed a thoracotomy on the day prior. For some reason, the nursing staff were feeding him on post-op day one, and all of sudden he started choking as I happened to walk into the room. He had gotten a piece of chicken caught in the larynx. I had them call the code, he sort of collapsed, and his saturations were falling. The intermediate level resident was out of the hospital, and the fellow was 12 floors below doing surgery. It was just me — all the nurses were just looking at me, like what do you want to do? I gave him a Heimlich maneuver to no avail. I gave him abdominal thrusts when he collapsed over on his side. At that point he had passed out, and I remember thinking, okay, just relax. For some reason that I cannot answer as it was a surgical ICU, the nurses could not find an endotracheal to attempt intubation. I used to carry a disposable scalpel in my pocket, so I made an incision in the cricothyroid membrane, which is not something an intern would be doing. Our intern class had learned it on a dog when we were accredited for critical care the week prior to starting our internship.

He ended up surviving and doing well, but it was a little hairy. With my faith, I was hoping that God was going to be with me. It is a little different when you have only done a procedure on a dog, but I felt like I was trained. Ultimately, I was glad when the intermediate resident and fellow showed up. That was a little nerve-wracking.

In hindsight, I thought, my gosh, what have I done. But I knew that it was the most appropriate thing — there was no tube to intubate the patient, and the next option was to try to bypass the blockage. I was later told by other attendings that I did the right thing. The worst thing I could have done would have been to sit there and be intimidated by the situation. After that day, I was proud that I hadn't shied away from the situation. But I was also very happy that the intermediate and fellow showed up, because they were more clinically experienced than I was.

What is it like being a chief resident?

There are three residents in our class, and we all function as chief residents. There is no selection of a chief resident. It is different from the intern year. We are responsible for teaching the junior residents on rounds. We essentially run the service as second- and third-year residents, but the chief resident makes the ultimate decisions. You get to spend more time in the operating room, and you have new responsibilities as the chief resident on the service. I spend more and more of my time reading about different surgical techniques and preparing for the operating room and less and less of my time returning pages from nursing staff. The attendings treat you almost as a colleague. They will ask you, "What will you do?" to see if there is something we are thinking that they haven't thought of.

What moments have been particularly meaningful as a chief resident?

I don't know if there's been one particular moment. Our year is rotated into four-month blocks, and on each rotation we are working with different attendings. I have enjoyed working with all the attendings. Our attendings give us a lot of respect, but they expect a lot of us. I enjoy that my opinion is valued, and I respect that they expect a lot out of us.

Who has been influential to you during your residency?

I have enjoyed each of our attendings at Loyola. However, the attendings that have motivated me the most are Dr. Turk, Dr. Quek, and Dr. Flanigan. Dr. Turk is one of those attendings that can be brutally honest when needed. I value constructive criticism, and I appreciate knowing his stance on my skills when we operate together. He also has a great knack for knowing when to intervene and when to watch during surgical cases. He really is the total package when I think of all the great qualities you want in a mentor.

Dr. Quek joined our faculty this year after finishing an oncology fellowship at USC. He has been an incredible mentor for me as I have watched how he has adjusted to being an attending. He has a great amount of patience with everyone in the hospital. Surgery has this misconception that you have to be arrogant to be a good surgeon. Dr. Quek is among the humblest surgeons I have met, yet he is also extremely talented.

Dr. Flanigan is our chairman. I have become impressed with his approach to resident education and making sure we get the appropriate number and mix of cases. He always tells us that we are like family to him. I can certainly vouch for this statement, as he is always interested in the residents' lives in and out of medicine. He will remain a close friend and mentor after my training at Loyola.

Do you feel confident of your ability to practice independently after graduation?

I do feel confident of my ability to practice independently. My philosophy is that as a physician you should be cognizant of your limits. When concerns arise, I will probably speak with prior attendings from Loyola to express concerns or to inquire about their surgical experience or expertise.

What are your plans after graduation?

I was accepted for a trauma/male reconstructive surgery fellowship at the University of California-San Francisco; however, it will not be until 2007–08. With an extra year before my fellowship in San Francisco, I was initially concerned about how I could fill this extra time. I remembered speaking with a physician in Chicago who had done an extra year in Australia after his training. I researched Australian fellowships and was eventually accepted for a one-year robotic and laparoscopic fellowship in Melbourne, Australia. Robotic surgery as a means to remove the prostate for prostate cancer has really exploded onto the urology scene in the past few years. Whether it stays or falls by the wayside remains to be seen; however, learning robotic surgery will be a useful surgical skill to have. It also won't hurt that I will be learning it in Australia for one year.

What advice would you give to medical school graduates starting their residencies?

I think my advice has changed since the 80-hour work rule came into effect [in July 2003]. There were negatives associated with it [residents being on duty more than 80 hours a week] but I feel more akin to teaching without the 80-hour work rule. It has kind of encouraged a lot of residents to take this philosophy of clocking in and clocking out. I would encourage junior residents to remember that there are days when you have to go the extra mile; there are days when you have to do things you don't want to do, but it's all for the patient. Going into medicine carries an extra responsibility that other professions don't have. You are putting the patients' care in your hands. When you go into private practice, you're not going to have the 80-hour rule. You have this incredible responsibility to take care of patients. It is not something to be endured, but to be enjoyed. There are a lot of people who would enjoy being in this situation where they can make an impact on someone else's life and not take it lightly.

You have to remain humble and remain cognizant of your limits. You should always be ready to ask for help, if needed, and not to think of consulting your colleagues as a sign of weakness. It is important to remember that as a physician, you are the same as the other people who work at your institution. Whether it's the operating room nurses, scrub techs, clinic nurses, or housekeepers, everyone wants to be treated with respect. As physicians, our jobs have additional responsibilities that are more vital, but in the end no one should walk around the hospital expecting to be treated like a god. Lastly, as a resident physician I always watch the attendings and how they treat their patients. As a result, I have learned better ways to console a patient, to handle difficult family situations, and to just listen to the patient even when I don't have the answers. The reflection of your personality is conveyed in how you treat your patients.

What is one thing that medicine does well and one thing that can be improved?

Your view as a resident is very naïve, because you don't have to deal with coding or insurance. From speaking to our attendings, I find this seems to be a very frustrating part of being a physician. It can cloud their reasons for going into medicine, especially the older physicians who have experienced the major changes in medicine over the last two decades. As a result many feel restricted because of the way medicine is run and don't enjoy the feeling of having power stripped from the control of the medical field. I don't know how this can be fixed. I don't have the answers. I guess this is just an observation of what medicine doesn't do well. I went to India for one week to perform urologic care during my chief resident year, and it was a completely different medical environment. The barrier to patient care seemed less intrusive, and all of the patients were so appreciative. It was an incredible opportunity for me to forget about all the negative intrusions into American medial care that can be frustrating and wearisome. In the end, it rekindled all the reasons why I chose to enter medicine. I hope to become involved with volunteer medical care as an attending, both for the underserved and for myself.

Sometimes the patient-physician relationship can be more difficult in the United States. For the most part, patients are very appreciative, but a lot of physicians have to practice defensive medicine because of the fear of being sued. No one enters the medical field with the mindset that he/she wants to do harm to patients. We walk a fine line in medicine where mistakes are not taken lightly. Patients want perfection, and sometimes it can be frustrating when your best effort is countered by a lawsuit. Patient quality of life for the rest of a person's life can be impacted positively or negatively by decisions that we will make. This is a tough pill to swallow initially as a young physician, but I think most all of us savor the chance to have this unique opportunity.

Is there anything else you'd like to say about your residency?

I enjoy the camaraderie of the residents. Our residency is small compared to the major medical fields with only three residents per year. Having such a small program allows everyone to get to know your habits — good and bad. People have asked, if you could do it all again, would you? Yes, definitely yes. There is an incredible sense of fulfillment that comes from being able to help people out. It is a big responsibility, and I look forward to becoming a better physician each year.

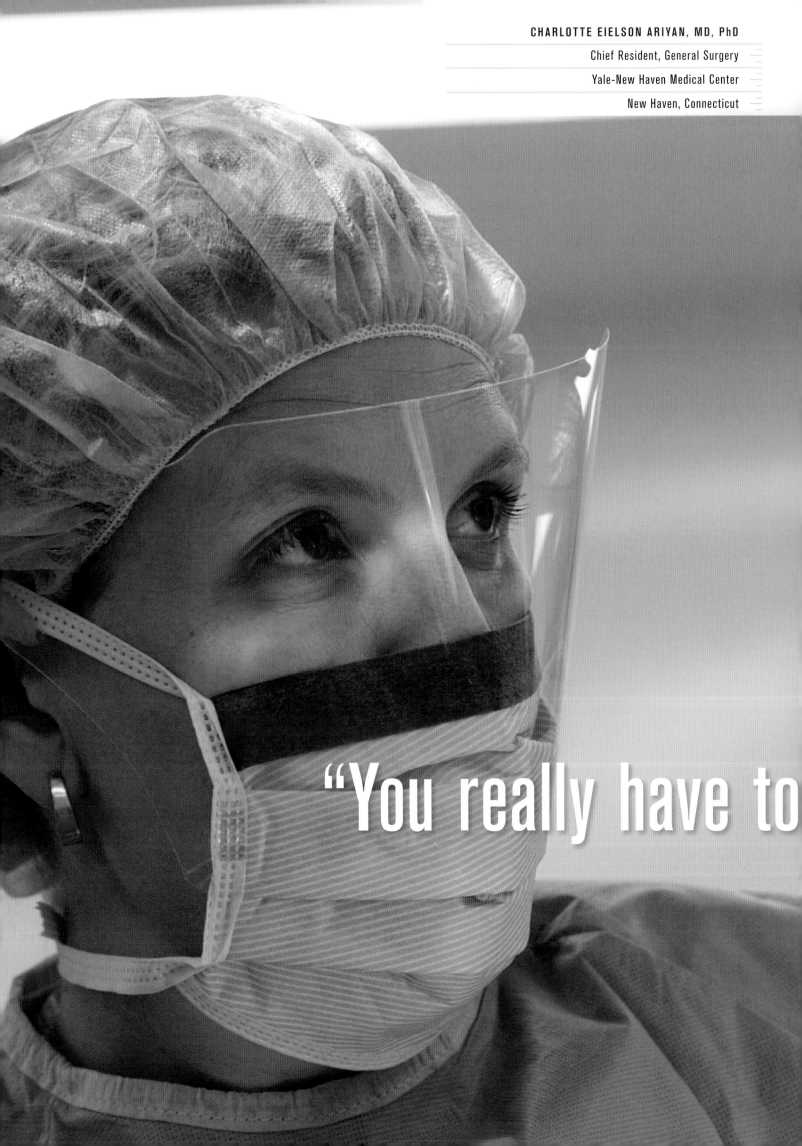

CHARLOTTE EIELSON ARIYAN, MD, PhD

Chief Resident, General Surgery

Yale-New Haven Medical Center

New Haven, Connecticut

"You really have to

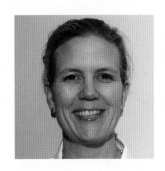

I f there is one thing that stands out for Charlotte Ariyan, MD, PhD, from her surgical residency at Yale-New Haven Medical Center, it is the mentors that have guided and taught her during her journey to become a surgeon. A mentor at the University of Vermont Medical School, where she earned her medical degree after graduating from the University of Connecticut with a dual undergraduate degree in neurobiology and Spanish, encouraged her interest in surgery. Faculty at Yale were also role models and teachers during her general surgery residency.

Dr. Ariyan, who also took a four-year break in her residency in order to earn a doctorate in philosophy and immunology from Yale, experienced many changes in her residency, including the introduction of the ACGME's common duty hour standards in 2003, the birth of her two children, and her own personal growth from an eager first-year resident to a confident and experienced chief resident.

Dr. Ariyan, who is married with two children, enjoys cooking, skiing, golfing and competing in triathlons.

How did you become interested in medicine and what attracted you to surgery?

I was always interested in surgery. I mean, always interested in medicine, I should say [laughs]. Even when I was young, I volunteered in a hospital. I liked science and thought it would be really great to go into medicine. Despite the fact that no one in my family was in medicine, my parents encouraged me, and I pursued this path.

think two steps ahead."

I went to medical school at the University of Vermont. The surgery department there is very strong and I had a lot of really great mentors. There were two people in particular, Dr. Shackford and Dr. Herbert, who set me on my career path and, in essence, changed my life. Before surgery I thought I would either do internal medicine or ob/gyn. Dr. Shackford was the chairman of surgery at UVM. He was a formidable character absolutely committed to excellence in medicine, family and fitness — he was an accomplished triathlete and marathoner. I also spent most of my daily time with Dr. Herbert, who was a less intense but brilliant surgeon who showed me the art of surgery. These were all things that I identified with. I felt like both Drs. Shackford and Herbert challenged people around them to rise to the occasion.

When I sat down to meet with Dr. Shackford and told him I was interested in surgery, he was so encouraging. He wrote me a personal letter, saying, "Charlotte, I am so happy to hear that you want to do surgery and I think you will go on to accomplish great things." I still have that letter to this day … it meant a lot to me.

During medical school, I completed an elective rotation at Yale and really enjoyed it. I met another wonderful mentor in New Haven, a vascular surgeon, Dr. Gusburg. I stayed in touch with him even after I finished doing my rotation. He was a gentle-mannered, great surgeon, who could distill any clinical or personal issue instantaneously. He is one of the best educators I have ever met. He offered me counsel on my career paths even after I returned to UVM to finish medical school. As I visited other potential general surgery residency programs, I thought, "Why would I go anywhere else when I know I can have such a great mentor at Yale?"

What were your feelings on the first day of your surgical residency?

When I first started my residency, one thing that was nice was that I was going to a place that was not completely new. I had done a rotation there and knew the place and the hospital … but I still remember being nervous and afraid and wanting to do a good job. And I was just so excited.

What was especially memorable about the first year of your residency?

When I look back on my first two years, we were working like crazy! I was often working on call every other night, and I was staying late during my post-call nights. The team worked closely resulting in memorable camaraderie among the residents. We relied on each other to survive. I knew everything about my patients. My life was the hospital, but it was a good time.

And now it is a completely different structure. That is the biggest thing that stands out between my internship and now: the structure of residency and training and how much it has changed. You hear some old-time surgeons say, "You know, it is not the way it used to be," but I can always respond, "Well, I started the way it used to be and now I am here, and I am a proponent of the new way" [laughs].

When you started your residency, did you feel confident that you would learn all that you needed to know?

The general surgery residency is five years in duration. It is a long time, and you know you are going to experience everything you need to see. The key, I think, is to extract as much as possible from each patient encounter because there is so much to learn from each patient.

Days are very structured in surgery. You round early, go to the operating room all day, and then round again. One day each week is spent in the clinic and doing academic activities, such as reviewing pathology and attending teaching conferences. In the operating room, there is always the attending. As the junior resident, you start going in and a lot of times you are just watching and slowly you start to do more things. So the bigger cases you sit in, the smaller stuff you get to gradually participate in, always with plenty of supervision. I never felt like I was left on my own by any means. I did not feel overwhelmed, but I think part of that was due to my experience as a medical student in Vermont; their medical student surgery track was very strong, and I definitely had the skills I needed when I left there: I knew how to suture, I knew how to tie knots, I was ACLS and ATLS certified. It gave me more confidence.

Why did you decide to get your PhD in immunology?

One of my earliest mentors at Yale was Dr. Bassadonna; he is a transplant surgeon who had a great immunology lab. Following year two of the surgery residency at Yale you are required to spend two years in the lab conducting research and publishing before completing your final three clinical training years. I started off in Dr. Bassadonna's lab and while there, Yale started an Investigative Medicine Program to provide a way for people who already have their MDs to get their PhDs. I thought it was such a great opportunity. Plus, Yale has a world-class immunology program, and the PhD would expand my time in the lab beyond a single person's lab and experience. Immunology transcends so many levels: organ transplantation, autoimmune diseases and oncology, which is actually what I plan to focus my career on now. I wanted to have more of an exposure to all aspects of immunology, so I applied and was accepted into Yale's PhD program.

Personally, it also gave me additional personal time. When I was in the lab, I got married and started a family toward the end of my lab time. It gave me opportunities to do those other things because I did not have to take a lot of call or have other clinical responsibilities.

I also had the opportunity to work at a hospice in Connecticut, which deals with people who are dying and at the end-stage of life. That was a very eye-opening experience for me. Medicine itself in the hospital is so focused on the data and the details of what is happening with the patient. And hospice is really the opposite — it is treating people's symptoms without a lot of data. You do not have monitors or a lot of diagnostics, so as a physician you depend much more on your clinical skills.

In medicine you see tragic stories all the time: someone gets into a car accident and dies and did not have any knowledge that he or she was going to die. But the people in hospice, in a way, have a gift because they know that they are going to die, and they have time to say the things and do the things they want/need to do. I admire their courage for being open to that. Also, I learned a lot professionally about how to talk to patients and their families, how to recognize when it really is the end, and what the symptoms are. Nowadays, there is more attention to that in the hospital, but when I first started, there really was not.

I am starting a surgical oncology fellowship at Memorial Sloan-Kettering, so being in hospice and working with these people was an experience I really felt I needed. Sometimes in surgery you are operating on people for palliative reasons to keep them comfortable and maintain their dignity, and you are not going to cure them. That is a tough discussion to have.

How did you grow personally and professionally throughout your residency?

When I was an intern, I came in as a person with fundamental knowledge and a skill set, but I was really someone collecting data, relaying information, and following directions. When you are an intern, your decisions are very small: little decisions about keeping people's electrolytes

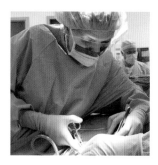 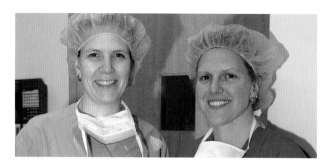

"THE DECISION-MAKING REALLY MAKES YOU A DIFFERENT PERSON."

in control, things like that. Then you become a chief, and you are still involved in all the small details, but you are really putting everything together into a much bigger picture. The biggest thing that comes through the whole transition during this time is that you really have to think two steps ahead as a chief and understand the implications of your decision and what that is going to mean. You are thinking about all the different ramifications, from small to big.

How is your chief residency the same as and different from the earlier years in your residency?

You transition from being a person that is taking care of a small domain to a person who is taking care of a very large domain. Of course, I have gained more technical and diagnostic skills since being an intern, but I think it is really the decision-making that makes you a different person.

We teach — you have a whole team of people, junior residents, medical students that work with you. You are responsible for them, which is definitely another change, too. In some ways it is more stressful because you are not only worried about all your patients, but also you are worried about your team and being able to provide feedback to people. It adds in a whole other level of complexity to being chief. And I think, as a chief, you want everyone to do well, and you want everyone to be happy and have those positive experiences the same way you did. So I feel a tremendous responsibility to help people along.

Has there been any moment in your chief resident year that has been particularly meaningful?

There are two things about chief year that are very rewarding. You are vested with all your patients and therefore you reap those rewards of seeing patients through the course, through their medical course — but also the rewards of the residents and the students that you get to work with, and you know, help them discover what their dreams are about. If they are interested in surgery, then that is special. I received two teaching awards from the students and the residents at Yale. That was a definite highlight for me.

What advice would you give to medical school graduates entering their residencies?

A lot of people do not know what they eventually want to specialize in, so I always encourage people to keep an open mind. But the biggest thing is to find a mentor, to find one early, because I think that is the biggest way to help a person through residency, which can be tough at times.

Throughout my chief year, my biggest mentor has been the program director, Dr. Walter Longo. He set the program back on track and taught me how to be an independent surgeon. As a chief you get to work with him very, very closely. I always say he is the best coach I ever had. He pushes you to be the best you can be, yet he is always there for you. He gave me the confidence I needed to perform well.

If you could improve one thing in medicine, what would it be, and what is one thing that you think medicine does particularly well?

The one thing that I think is difficult, unfortunately, is the business side to medicine now. In our training, we do not get involved in the business aspect of medicine. Rather, our focus is on learning to diagnosis and treat clinically. But the bottom line is, you come out of training and you have to deal with the insurance companies and deal with all these different types of payments. This is a stressor for the patients as well. We need to get some more formalized education on the different types of insurance, how to bill, collect, appeals process, etc.

Also, so many medical students are graduating with over $100,000 of debt. That is hard because it is influencing what people are going to do and how much time they are willing to spend in training. The system desperately needs to find a way to decrease the cost of medical education. Increasingly, would-be, future, talented physicians are deciding to go to law and business school, which only requires a two-to three-year commitment with less debt and often lucrative starting salaries.

Residency programs are great forums for really training doctors and giving them a complete picture on what it means to be a physician. I think that is why people come from other countries around the world to the United States to have that opportunity. It is not that we have the most unusual diseases here; it is just that we are really able to provide that forum of sharing and education.

Is there anything else that you would like to say about your residency?

As I mentioned earlier, the biggest thing for me was my mentors throughout medical school and residency. That was really important to me. The other thing is the camaraderie that I felt among my fellow residents — friendships that I will take with me for a lifetime. They were a wonderful support. I also was lucky. In medical school, there were other women who went into surgery. One was my best friend, Jackie Jeruss. She went through the general surgery program at Northwestern in Chicago. She also got her PhD, is married and has kids. We have been in tandem every step of the way since our time in medical school at the University of Vermont. It has been a real gift to have a friend like that, someone who knows first hand the ups-and-downs that you experience, professionally and personally, every day.

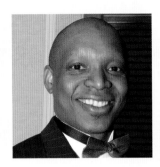

*A*s a child growing up in Belize, Dr. Clifford Perez, MD, didn't dream that one day he would be working as a surgeon in Nebraska. A scholarship gave him the opportunity to come to the United States and attend college. After receiving degrees in mathematics and biology from Minnesota State University, Dr. Perez taught in a high school in Belize for two years before returning to the United States and enlisting in the U.S. Air Force. He earned his medical degree from the Medical University of South Carolina in Charleston. He completed a one-year internship at the Mayo Medical Clinic in Rochester, Minnesota, and then did research in surgical nutrition at Harvard University for two years before beginning his surgical residency at Creighton University Medical Center, where he was a chief resident in 2005–06.

After graduation, Dr. Perez began active duty as a major with the U.S. Air Force, serving at Travis Air Force Base in Fairfield, California. Dr. Perez relaxes by spending time with his family, exercising and reading.

Why did you decide to become a doctor?

I am the sixth of 11 kids. I was born in a small town, Belmoden, in Belize. I moved here as a teenager to go to college. Nine other Belizians received the same scholarship to go to Minnesota State University, so I was not exactly alone. It was, however, leaving my family since we are close-knit and I saw myself as one of the providers. There was the initial culture shock because I moved from someplace warm to someplace cold!

From my late teens I had been interested in medicine. I always wanted to do some service-related job, and medicine seemed to be the perfect fit.

"*Choose a residency that*

Why did you choose Creighton for your residency?

My mentor at the time was a general surgeon, Dr. Danny Jacobs, here at Creighton. He is African-American, and he was the chairman of the program. I met him at Brigham and Women's Hospital. I often refer to his advice "to work hard and never let them see you sweat." I understood this to remain unflappable and to maintain my competency in the face of adversity.

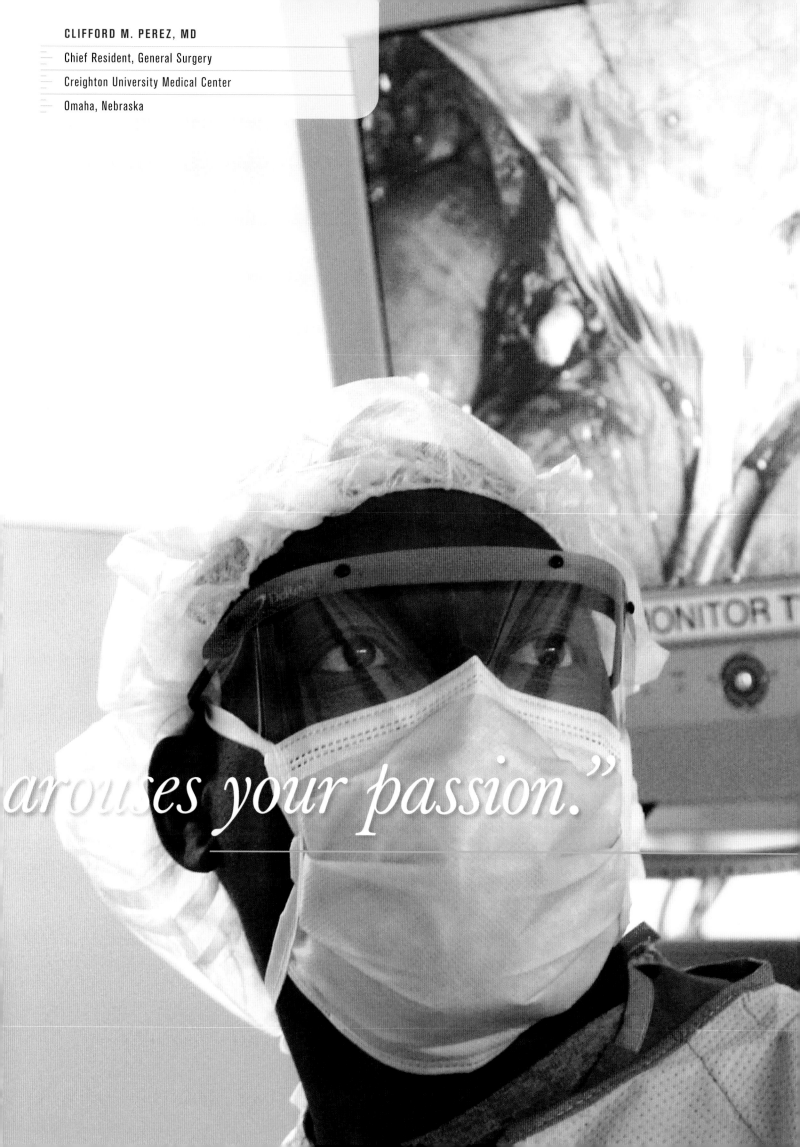

CLIFFORD M. PEREZ, MD

Chief Resident, General Surgery

Creighton University Medical Center

Omaha, Nebraska

arouses your passion."

What stands out from the first year of your residency?

I definitely felt that it was going to be challenging, but I thought I would be able to learn enough to handle whatever challenges there were. I was pretty enthusiastic and energetic. My first night on call was pretty terrifying; I was worried there would be a situation that I couldn't handle. But I became less nervous. I found out you are not alone as a physician. There are always people in residency training who have more knowledge than you.

My first night on call, I had an orthopedic surgery patient who went into alcohol withdrawal, and I remember the nurses helping me to manage him. Then I remember some of the people who I was taking care of who eventually died as a result of ailments they had. I felt sad, especially since I was very attached to the patients. I took it hard the first couple of times. I wondered if there was something else that could have been done to help them. I am a pretty spiritual person, and I feel that some people have the capacity within themselves to survive horrendous things, and somehow we assist and facilitate, but we can't take all the credit for the success. You can just do the best you can do with the knowledge that you have.

What is it like being a chief resident?

Everyone is a chief resident in their final year. It's not something you compete for. Your knowledge and technical skills are such that you are given more responsibilities to become independent as a surgeon. The way you are treated by the attending surgeons is definitely different as a chief resident. They tend to be more willing to impart some of their technical skills to you that they know you will need to practice. They also give you more responsibility and more autonomy in terms of decision-making, and also with minor surgical procedures that you can accomplish on your own. As chief resident you are essentially in charge of your patients. You are their surgeon, you evaluate them clinically, you treat them surgically, you take care of them post-operatively. You are responsible for organizing some of the educational activities, and also responsible for organizing the call schedule. We also help troubleshoot things and serve as liaisons between the residents and the attendings. I find it very rewarding. If I can impart to others whatever experience I have and make their education more meaningful, I like that role.

What is a typical day as a chief resident like?

Early in the morning, around 5 or 5:30, I see all my patients before surgery starts, and then surgery gets going in early morning. Some days we have a conference that starts early in the morning. I go on to do the surgery itself when we have cases to do. At the end of the day, when all of our cases are completed, I spend additional time going back and looking at patients who may have had particular problems. I do a post-op check. So I have fairly long days — they start at 5 a.m. and end at 7 p.m. Of course, when I get home, there is usually reading to do.

The 80-hour duty hour standard has psychologically made a big change. When you are on call, even if you have a very busy call night, you get to go home and take a break and come back again. Psychologically, that is good, but at times you feel like you miss out on continuity of patient care. Surgery is not a typical nine-to-five job. In surgery, you may be taking care of a patient, and then the 80-hour limit is up, and you have to turn over that care to someone else. But, psychologically, the 80-hour limit is good. It acknowledges that you are human and have limits to functioning effectively. It gives you an opportunity to take a break, as opposed to being this macho physician. You don't feel bad about saying "I am tired."

How have you grown professionally and personally during your residency?

I have grown more confident in my technical and clinical skills. I have become more aware of my limitations as a physician and a surgeon. I've become more cautious and aware of the impact that we have on people's lives. I was more impulsive as a student clinician. Now I am less impulsive and more likely to be patient and work things out.

I am more humble. Being a physician or a surgeon doesn't make you any more special than another individual.

What advice would you give medical school graduates who are starting their residencies?

Choose a residency that arouses your passion and makes you want to get up and go to work every day. Your heart is the most important organ because if you love your patients, you will be motivated to study and work hard on their behalf.

Keep things in perspective. Residency is like boot camp. It is not the real world, and it ends.

What are your career plans?

My plans are to make the military a career. One of the things I like about it is that it seems to be like a social service; you are treating people who need treatment. You are not doing it for financial gain.

What does medicine do well and what do you think needs to be improved?

What works well is the apprenticeship-type training, where you grow in your responsibilities through mentorship.

What could be improved is the cost of medical education. If medical education was less expensive, then it would tend to attract people who aren't shooting for specialties that will earn them a lot of money so they can pay off their medical school debt. I would link medical education with service. For instance, the military assisted me with my education and now I have to give them my service.

I am married and have two children; I got married just before my residency. My wife is a nurse practitioner. It was very difficult to balance being a good parent and a good husband and maximize my energy for training. I draw inspiration from my sisters because they are single parents, and they haven't had the opportunities that I have had. Whatever difficulties I have, I compare myself to them, and they have had even greater obstacles to overcome.

90   96   100   108

 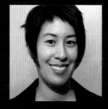 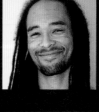 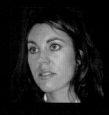

 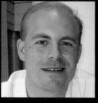 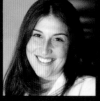

114   118   124

SPECIALISTS

"At some point I realized that learning
is a continuous process, and that this is
just the beginning."

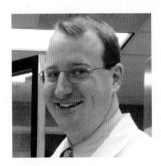

*A*s an undergraduate student majoring in liberal arts at Thomas Aquinas College in Santa Paula, California, Sam Caughron, MD, wasn't sure what career he wanted to pursue, but he knew he wanted to be in a service-oriented profession. Although Dr. Caughron founded his own software company while still in college, his father was a pathologist, which piqued his interest in medicine. Dr. Caughron completed his medical degree in 2002 at Creighton University School of Medicine and then entered the pathology residency program at Creighton University Medical Center. He served as chief resident in 2005–06.

In July 2006, Dr. Caughron began a fellowship in molecular pathology at Vanderbilt University in Nashville. Dr. Caughron is married and has six children. In his spare time, Dr. Caughron works as CEO of his small software company, studies for his private pilot's license and enjoys spending time with his family.

What made you interested in medicine?

I grew up in rural Kansas City, then attended undergraduate college at Thomas Aquinas College in southern California. It was liberal arts with a lot of theology and philosophy. I graduated with a sense of wanting to do something that is service-oriented. A lot of teachers come out of that school, but I chose medicine. My dad is also a physician; he is a pathologist, and so that was something I had some experience with. That is what originally turned me toward medicine. I was not, I guess, a typical medical student in that I wasn't aiming for it from day one. It was more that I thought I'd give it a go and see if I could get in, and if I did, I would see that as a calling to serve others. At the same time, I had done a lot of IT and software development work and started a company and had some software that was commercially published that I was selling. So I chose medicine. I didn't fall into it.

"THE BUCK STOPS HERE,

I came to Creighton University for medical school because it was here in the Midwest, it has a good reputation, and it is a Catholic school. I did my medical training here and chose to stay on for my residency in pathology as well. Next year I will be going to Vanderbilt in Nashville for a fellowship in molecular pathology. I entered medical school thinking I would go into primary care, and then I found that pathology was a better fit for my personality. I like the analytical aspects of pathology; also pathology tends to be the final authority on some issues. We can

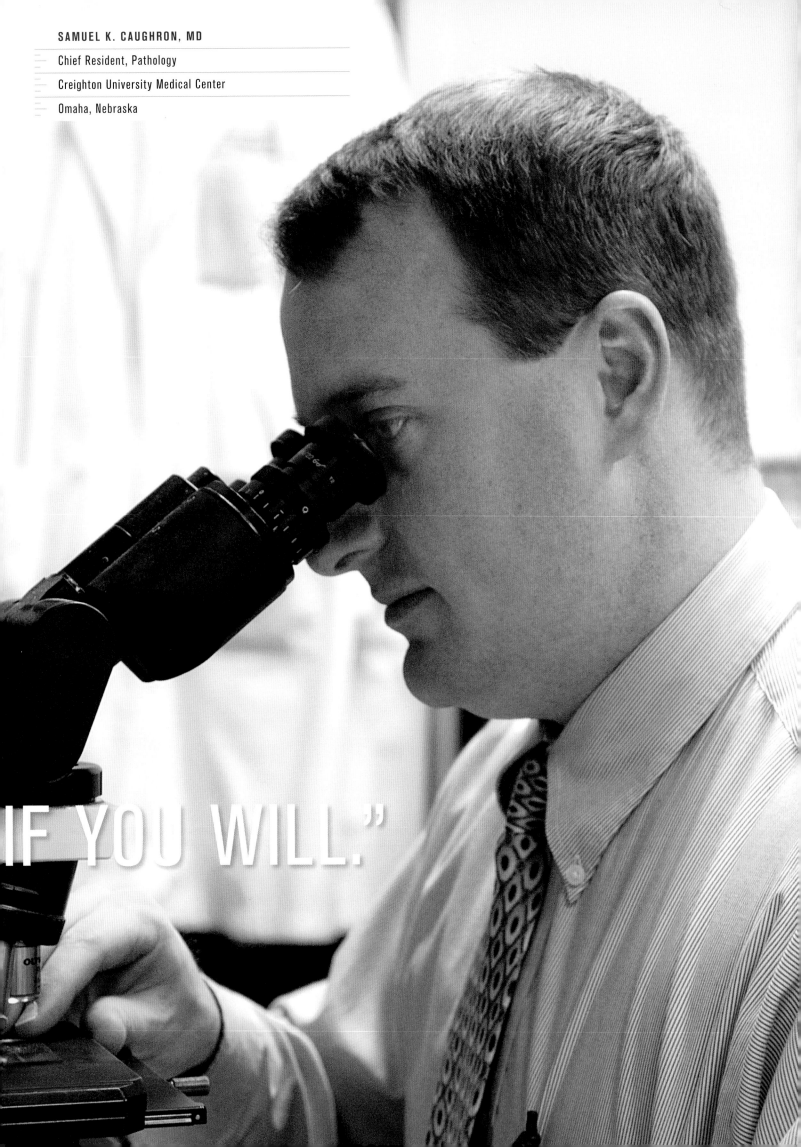

SAMUEL K. CAUGHRON, MD

Chief Resident, Pathology

Creighton University Medical Center

Omaha, Nebraska

IF YOU WILL."

refer to other pathologists, but the buck stops here, if you will. We get to see the interesting cases whether it is tissue or blood or specimens. If we can't answer it, there probably isn't an answer. I enjoy having that final say, if you will. I also enjoy the fact that I spend a lot of time interacting with my fellow physicians. We exist to support those who are seeing patients, and that means we interact with them quite a bit, and that is very rewarding to me.

Describe the first day of your residency.

Within the day-to-day routine, we spend a large portion of time looking at the specimens that are coming from surgery and the doctor's office and making the diagnosis of cancer or whatever else you may find to help your clinical colleagues. My first day, I showed up in my pressed white, now-long coat, instead of a short coat. I was very excited and optimistic about things and a little bit proud to finally be wearing that white coat and have that MD after my name and be doing what I had trained for four years to do, and also was a little bit afraid. There's just a huge unknown, and you know that now you are the one who is expected to give the final answer, so there is a little bit of trepidation.

Within my first month, I was very busy. Going into pathology I had expected things to be not as difficult as internships in other specialties. In this I was mistaken, and I remember towards the end of my first month going to my program director and telling him I felt overwhelmed and that I knew I was a very capable individual, but that the system must somehow be broken because as a capable individual I was feeling overwhelmed. He consoled me and reassured me and told me that was fairly common and to push on and things would get better, and sure enough, they did. That was a new experience for me to feel overwhelmed. In medical school you go through a lot, but it's on a different level once you get into your actual residency.

"THERE'S JUST A HUGE UNKNOWN, AND YOU KNOW THAT NOW YOU ARE THE ONE WHO IS EXPECTED TO GIVE THE FINAL ANSWER."

The second moment that stands out [in the first year] is that at most hospitals there is a tumor conference where the pathologists meet with surgeons and radiologists to discuss interesting cases. My first month, I was in the hot seat. I was told that I would be presenting the cases in front of the entire surgery department and was a little bit cautious and fearful of the situation. I remember a more senior pathologist telling me that although I had only had three weeks of pathology, I probably already knew more looking through the microscope than all of the surgeons in the room. Looking back on it, it was probably true. It speaks to the difference in what we do as pathologists and the value of the service we provide. It really does require a different professional level of skills that you don't find in the other areas of medicine. I did okay. I kind of made things up, I knew the basics, I had been a medical student a month ago, I sort of mumbled through and said some things I had heard the other pathologists say and none of the surgeons seemed to know that I didn't know what I was talking about. That's when I sort of realized — as I went through my training, I did come to know what I was talking about — that pathologists provide a service that is invaluable to the rest of the specialties.

What is your chief resident year like? How is it different from and the same as your first year?

There are always two chief residents. In my case, because of how the other residents were arranged, I sort of fell into the opportunity. In a way, the chief residency is a very difficult position because everyone below you sees you as being at the top and you should be able to make things better, and everyone above you sees you as responsible for making things better, so you are kind of caught in this squeeze from the top and bottom and everything gets pitched to you.

In pathology you do the same thing every year of your training. The duties are the same for the most part. But the level and autonomy that you accomplish them with change dramatically. So on a daily basis, the slides come out that are made from the tissue the lab receives. As a first year resident, I would look at them and try to figure out what the tissue was, and now as a chief I look at them and render a complete report, and the faculty just signs off on it, so there is a pretty significant difference in terms of professional competence.

Personally, there is a huge difference of growth. Residency is the time really when you become a doctor. You start out as a doctor, but you don't see yourself as a doctor. For a lot of people, that first year of internship is when you sort of see yourself as a doctor, and you develop the habits of thinking, the confidence in yourself, to really trust yourself with someone else's well-being. So as a chief resident, personally, that is a huge difference. I now see myself as a fellow pathologist and as a colleague to all physicians in the care of patients. No longer am I underneath them, but now I sort of stand shoulder to shoulder with them.

There was a case we had my second year that we presented at a thoracic oncology conference. I had seen the case and reviewed it with the faculty. We went to the conference to discuss it with the other thoracic surgeons and the pulmonologists. I remember disagreeing with my staff in that I wanted to call it a malignancy, where they were not as sure. And we presented the case and subsequently they did a resection of the patient's lung, and it came back that it was indeed a malignancy. That stands out in my mind because I had actually contributed something individually that was right and made a difference in the patient's care. I don't know if that was a turning point, but that sort of typifies the changes that happened.

Who was most influential to you during your residency?

Two people stood out for me; well, actually two people and a group of people. The first was my father. I didn't appreciate it at the time, but he has been something of a mentor to me in terms of being a more senior doctor that I can talk to about any questions I have. The other person was my residency director. Here at Creighton we are blessed to have a wonderful individual, William Hunter, MD, who believes in the residents. He is willing to let us go out on a limb, willing to let us make mistakes, yet sort of gently oversees us and make sure we don't get into too much hot water. He has been an incredible asset to my training.

The other group that I would mention is, as a pathologist, interacting with the clinicians. It is a little unique in pathology as a resident because you are immediately interacting with all the staff and faculty. When we have something to convey to the team, we will frequently call the staff rather than the resident. That opportunity to interact with them has meant a lot to me.

I am blessed to have the most wonderful woman in the world for my wife. I really couldn't have done it without her. Having a full personal life has been a source of great support for me. When I leave the hospital, there is a fullness there and meaning in life that keeps me focused on what is really important. When I go back, I am able to attack my job with greater strength and commitment, I guess. It gives meaning to what I do. Not only am I working for the sake of the patient, but also working to provide for and be an example to my family. That is something that I don't think everyone has, but it really is a huge benefit to those who do have it.

What advice would you give to medical school graduates entering their residencies?

I guess believe in yourself. It is easy that first year to have your confidence shaken. You certainly need to listen to those who are more senior to you, but also keep a critical mind because already you have a lot to contribute. There's a lot to learn, but even as a starting resident you have a lot to contribute. Believe in yourself and believe in your ability to contribute and don't forget that you've gone through medical school and the tough times. You have made the cut and you are up to the tough job you have in front of you.

If you could change one thing in medicine, what would that be?

Maybe it is just being a chief resident, but there is so much focus on the administrative aspect. It seems like the health system has lost focus on the patient-physician relationship. And fortunately, that still is preserved every day in the interactions that take place. But with cost-cutting, there are so many constraints on the system. It would nice to see a refocus within medicine on physicians providing not just the best health care, but really providing the health care that the individual needs. It's almost a holistic approach, if that makes any sense. I guess it's been a little disillusioning to see how much the administrative, insurance-related issues, cost issues, are a part of medicine. It would nice to see the system restructured somehow that those were not so much a focus.

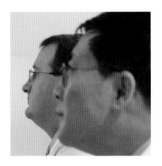 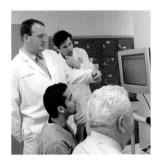 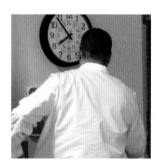

"RESIDENCY IS THE TIME REALLY WHEN YOU BECOME A DOCTOR."

What works well in medicine?

Advances that are being made technically are just incredible. Our ability to detect cancers earlier will become dramatic, our ability to treat cancer earlier and with fewer side effects will improve dramatically. The tools of the trade are at an incredible level now and are going to accelerate over the next ten years. Having those tools means that the quality of health care being delivered has improved in the last several years and is going to continually improve. In that context, the physician-patient relationship needs to be preserved. I attended a conference in Washington, DC, with high level government and insurance individuals. There was a lot of talk of individualized medicine and re-empowering the patients to take control of their health care which I think overall is a good thing. But what may be lost, which is actually what originally attracted me to medicine, is the notion of the town doctor who knows the patients, knows more than just a chart, and takes care of them in a complete way.

Any other thoughts on your residency?

There are a lot of physicians these days who are jaded because medicine has changed a lot. I've run into physicians who will advise people not to go into medicine, but I guess as someone who chose to go into medicine and had other opportunities, I don't regret it at all. As long as you remember the fundamental opportunity and honor it is to help others in a very personal way, it is extremely rewarding. So don't listen to the naysayers.

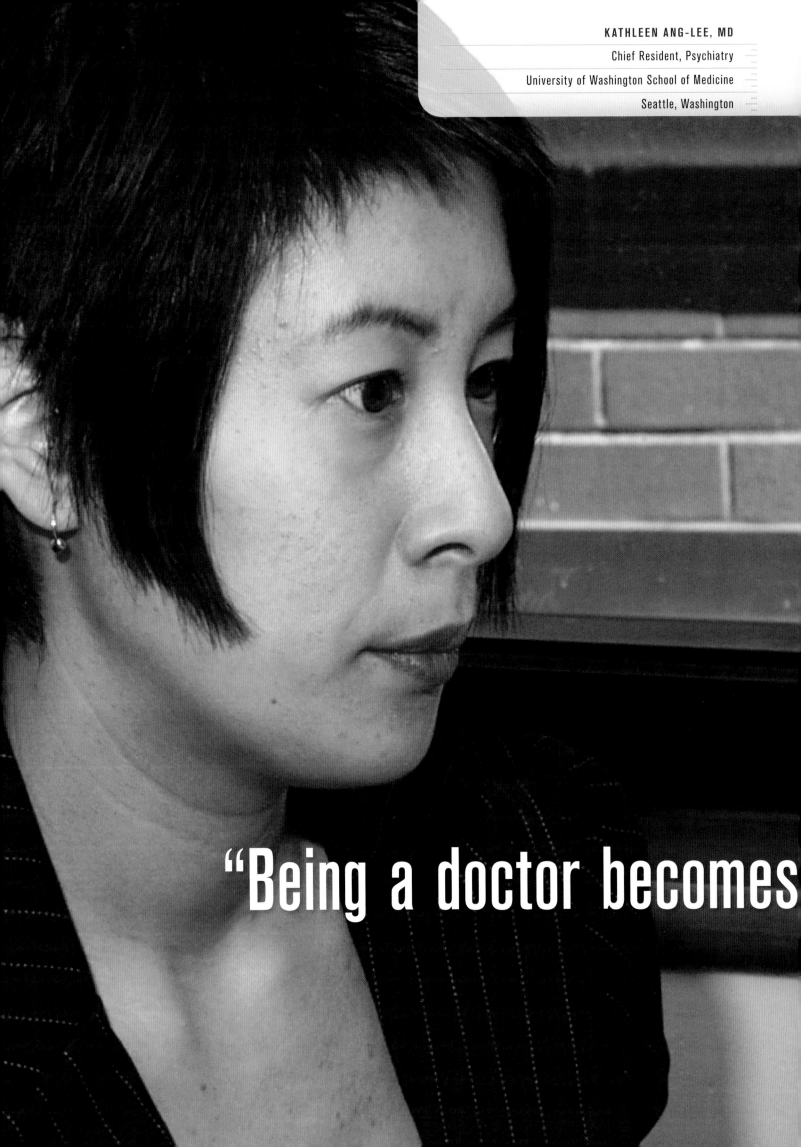

KATHLEEN ANG-LEE, MD

Chief Resident, Psychiatry

University of Washington School of Medicine

Seattle, Washington

"Being a doctor becomes

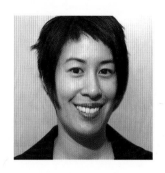

I t was the encouragement of Kathleen Ang-Lee's own physician, David C. Leach, MD, that helped her choose a career in medicine. After graduating from the University of Michigan in 1996, Dr. Ang-Lee completed her medical degree at the University of Chicago Pritzker School of Medicine. She discovered that it was the patients' stories that most interested her, and she decided to become a psychiatrist. During her residency, Dr. Ang-Lee contributed a chapter on psychiatry for a book on choosing a medical specialty. She served as the chief resident at the University of Washington Outpatient Psychiatry Clinic in 2005–06.

Dr. Ang-Lee is continuing her training in the University of Washington with an addiction psychiatry fellowship and plans on specializing in treating women with addictions. In her spare time, Dr. Ang-Lee, who is married with one child, enjoys cooking and travel.

Why did you decide to go into medicine?

I do not think I can overestimate the importance of role models in physicians' career decisions. Even though my parents are not physicians, they both work in science-related fields and have always encouraged my interest in science. We would perform science experiments in the kitchen together and I would often visit my mother at work in her lab. Medicine seemed a good way to integrate this interest with working with people. Additionally, Dr. David Leach was my physician when I was in high school. He was very supportive of my interest in medicine and even gave me his personal copy of *Harrison's Internal Medicine.* His encouragement meant a lot to me.

What made you choose psychiatry?

In medical school, I found that I most enjoyed hearing patients' stories and trying to understand how and why people feel and behave the way that they do. This is one of the last true mysteries of the human body. It is a very exciting time to be in psychiatry, especially given the rapid developments in neuroscience.

incorporated into who you are."

Deciding on a specialty was the easy part for me. The more difficult part was deciding on which residency programs I wanted to apply to. The University of Washington psychiatry residency program ended up as my first choice. It seemed to provide excellent training while at the same time had happy residents. In my opinion, the most important indicator of a program's quality is the attitude of the residents. If they are not happy, you can see it in their eyes even if they tell you otherwise.

What was your first day of residency like?

It was equal parts excitement and fear. I was excited to actually start practicing medicine after what seemed like an eternity as a student. During the last three months of medical school, I was itching to take responsibility for patients. However, once I got that responsibility on the first day of residency, I was afraid of not knowing enough and had nightmares of hurting a patient through my inexperience. Part of my first day included an orientation by the chief resident, and I quickly realized that I could rely on the chief resident for support. Over time, my confidence grew, and I learned quickly because the learning curve when you first start residency is so huge.

Is there any moment that stands out from that first year?

I will always remember the first time a patient called me "doctor." At first, I did not even realize that she was addressing *me*. It took me a while before I felt comfortable introducing myself as "Doctor Ang-Lee"! There are plenty of other moments from my first year as well … watching my first floridly manic patient return to baseline after weeks of treatment … the first time I performed ECT … the first time I had to go to court to try to keep an involuntarily committed patient who needed treatment from leaving … and of course, many, many long call nights.

How have you grown professionally and personally throughout your residency?

I have grown a lot through my contact with patients, colleagues and mentors. Residency has definitely broadened my outlook on medicine and life. With the growth in knowledge and clinical skill, my confidence in my abilities has grown as well. At some point, being a doctor becomes incorporated into who you are. It becomes a part of your identity.

I am lucky in that my husband has been very supportive in my residency. He is an anesthesiologist working in private practice. Through him, I have seen the business side of medicine they never teach you in residency, since he has been quite busy helping to run his group practice.

How is the chief resident year different from the first year?

This year is completely different from my first year because I am in a leadership position now. As a chief resident, I have to balance administrative and clinical duties. In psychiatry, serving as a chief resident is not an additional year as it is in some other specialties. I am one of five chiefs, one for each of our clinical sites.

Who was most influential to you during your residency?

There are definitely a lot of people. My program director, Deborah Cowley, MD, who received the ACGME's Parker J. Palmer Courage to Teach award, has been an inspiration and support to all of us in the residency. She is a role model and a great psychiatrist.

My mentor in addiction psychiatry, Andrew Saxon, MD, has been my preceptor over my four years and has provided me with research opportunities. One of my fondest memories of residency is spending Fridays in an addictions research group with two other friends of mine in the residency.

My residency class also has a T-group. It meets once a week and is an open forum for us to discuss issues that come up in residency or our personal lives. My T-group leader, Rick Adamson, MD, is a private practitioner who volunteers his time. He has been very influential in providing support via T-group and has also been a mentor to several of us who are interested in private practice.

Are there any moments from your chief residency that stand out?

Meeting the new interns at their orientation and giving them a talk about surviving call and surviving internship. It was the first time my role shifted from being the student to the teacher. It was gratifying to help them out in their first anxious days. It was also nice to see how far I had come from being an intern at that time.

When did you start thinking of yourself as a doctor?

It is hard to pinpoint the exact moment — sometime in my intern year when I started feeling more confident in managing my patients. Another major shift occurred in my third year of residency, when I switched from working in an inpatient setting to outpatient clinics. I started developing long-term relations with patients and began learning more about psychotherapy.

What advice would you give to medical school graduates?

I would advise them to just try to get as much out of the residency as they can. It is the only time you will be able to do something outside of your comfort zone and have an attending there to back you up. Keep an open mind throughout your training. Stay interested in everything and find opportunities to learn everywhere. You would be surprise how you end up using little tidbits of knowledge from rotations you never even considered. Learning does not end with medical school or residency. I would also advise them to take care of themselves as well, because residency, especially internship, can be quite grueling at times — both physically and emotionally.

If you could change one thing about medicine, what would that be?

I would like to see the end of the stigma of mental health, improve the disparity in the health care system in the United States and have more mental health parity. I would also like to see a reduction in the litigious culture that forces physicians to practice defensive, and sometimes unnecessary, medicine. I think it is something that all physicians have to worry about.

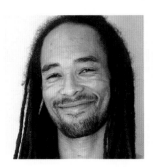

R obert J. Gore, MD, was still in high school when he decided to become a physician. However, he was determined not to let his career overshadow his other interests. As an undergraduate at Morehouse College in Atlanta, he took a broad range of liberal arts classes in addition to his pre-med courses. During his years of medical school at the State University of New York at Buffalo and his residency at Cook County Hospital, he continued to pursue his interests in photography, travel and martial arts. He recently spent time in Peru for an elective in emergency medicine.

Dr. Gore also serves as a mentor to African-American students who are thinking of careers in medicine and often invites them to spend a day with him at the hospital.

After graduation, Dr. Gore began working as an attending physician at Kings County Hospital in Brooklyn, New York.

Why did you become interested in medicine?

I grew up in Brooklyn, New York. My junior year of high school, I was training for cross country and I got injured. I had to go see an orthopedic surgeon. The orthopedic surgeon kind of became my mentor, and my interest sparked from that point on.

"I felt like this is where

I went to Morehouse College in Atlanta. Morehouse was a unique experience, because it is an historically black college, but it is also all-male, and it is a liberal arts college. It is the only institution in the United States geared toward educating black males. In that environment we had a number of different mentors that took an active role in making sure that we succeeded and became physicians; it was something that was stressed from the first day. We had a pre-med adviser, a guy by the name of Dean Blocker, and he got all the freshmen who were interested in medicine or the sciences together during the first two weeks of school and he said, "This is what you guys need to do in order to get into medical school or to get your PhDs," so we pretty much kept on track for that four-year period. But it was a liberal arts school, so music was stressed, philosophy was stressed, and we had to take courses in sociology and public speaking, just to make us more well-rounded students.

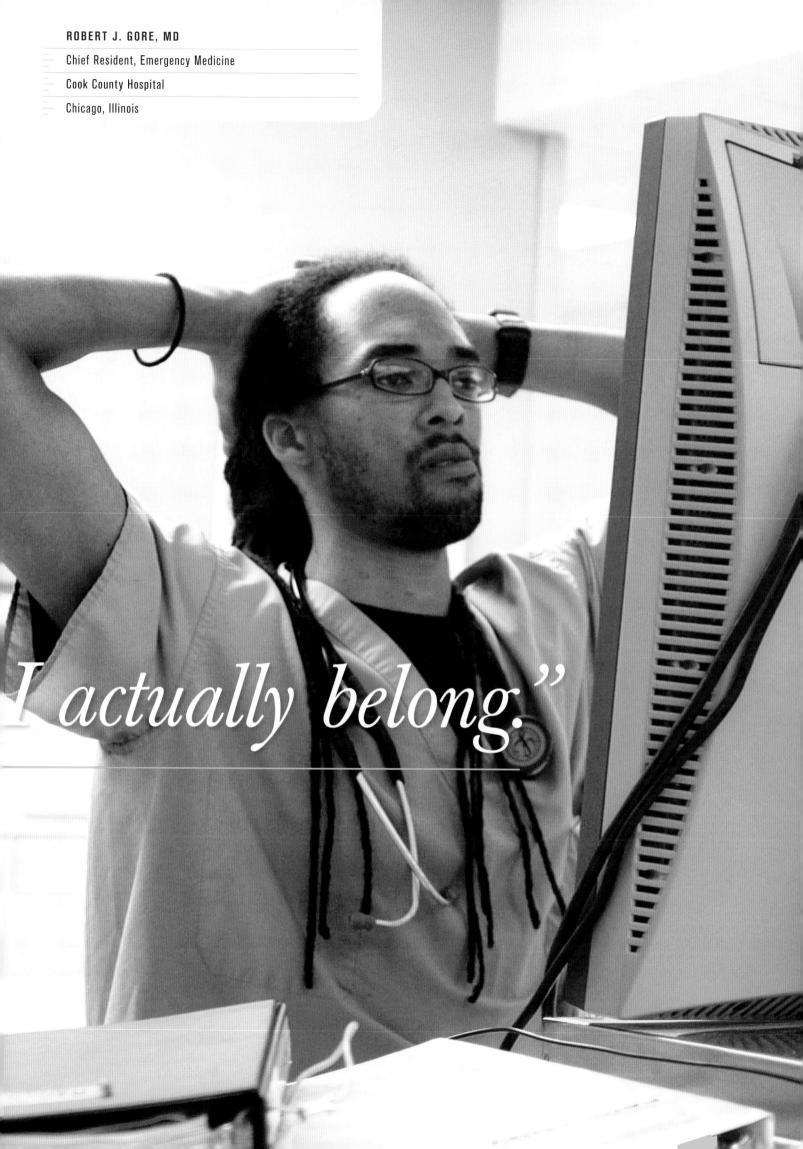

ROBERT J. GORE, MD

Chief Resident, Emergency Medicine

Cook County Hospital

Chicago, Illinois

I actually belong."

I still read actively, I still partake in other interests. I think it makes you a more complete being, as opposed to being someone who is so one-dimensional that you cannot relate to anything else around you. It is extremely important when it comes to taking care of patients. In emergency medicine we take care of people from all walks of life and all ages, and some of the experiences that you have in college, from reading on different cultures and studying those different cultures and learning how other people think and work, helps us establish a quick rapport with our patients.

What interested you about emergency medicine?

That is also interesting. I initially thought that I was going to go into sports medicine. Later on, that interest changed into pediatrics. During third year, I did internal medicine first. I really enjoyed that, but I could not see myself doing that every day. I did psychiatry, loved it. After seven weeks I said to myself, "I do not think I can do this every day but I can apply this no matter what I do." When I did surgery, things started to kind of click. I was able to work with my hands for the very first time, and enjoyed the experience. A friend of mine said, "Why don't you just do emergency medicine?" I said, "Get out of here, I cannot do that." But I did a rotation in the emergency department and for the first time in three years — actually three and a half years — I felt like this is where I actually belong. The residents kind of had that same philosophy with their overall outlook on life. They had multiple interests, they were involved in many different hobbies and that really sounded like me. I felt really comfortable being in the emergency department and decided to apply for an emergency residency program.

Cook County was my top choice. I knew that I wanted to work in a public hospital in a major urban area. I went to medical school in Buffalo, which is urban, but it is not a very large city. I also rotated in Kings County Hospital in New York City, which is where I am going to be an attending. I had an excellent experience there as a medical student but realized that I needed to get out of Brooklyn. I had relatives in Chicago, and I heard a lot of good things about Cook County's program, and I interviewed and I enjoyed it.

I did my internship at Cook County Hospital, part of the old hospital, which was an interesting experience [laughs]. I got a pretty good foundation in internal medicine, as well as some exposure to some of the specialties. All of the stuff is done to help supplement your experience when you start your emergency medicine program.

What were you feeling when you first started your internship year?

Fear [laughs]. We have a natural fear of the unknown. Medical students, physicians, residents — many of us are perfectionists. A lot of us have these Type A personalities and feel like you have to know everything. When someone calls you "Doctor" for the first time, you feel like you have this sense of responsibility. Which is important; I think you should feel like you have a major responsibility. However, early on, you feel like you have to know everything. The nurses are going to ask you questions, your patients are going to ask you questions, you have questions about specific situations relating to your patients in the hospital. And if you do not know the answer, sometimes it can be nerve-wracking.

One thing that I came to realize is that everybody else, every other physician, has gone through what you have gone through, and they expect you to ask for help. They do not expect you to know everything, and you should not expect yourself to know everything. The people who do not ask for help, I think, are always the ones who make the most mistakes.

As a matter of fact, most attendings — even your senior-most attendings — do not have all the answers. And they are the first people to say, "Okay, well, I am going to go look this up, because I do not have a freaking clue what this is." And I think that makes us feel a little bit more comfortable, and say, "Okay, I do not have to have all the answers for this specific situation."

Is there anything that stands out from the first year of your residency?

It was probably the second day of my internship. I was on a cardiology consult and I went to see a patient to pre-op him. I went to introduce myself. I said, "Hi, I am Dr. Gore, I am one of the interns, I am going to be taking care of you." And the guy started to cry. And I said, "Uh oh. Why is he crying?" This is my second day of residency. I am not used to seeing guys cry, and it did get a little uncomfortable for me. And I got him a tissue and was like, you know, "Are you okay, sir?" And he says, "You do not understand." I said, "What?" "I am so proud of you." And I said, [laughs], "You are? I want to know why are you crying?" He says, "You know, I have never had a black physician before and seeing what you are doing right now makes me so proud."

"THE PEOPLE WHO DO NOT ASK FOR HELP, I THINK, ARE ALWAYS THE ONES WHO MAKE THE MOST MISTAKES."

It gave me another boost of confidence. This was my second day of someone calling me "Doctor." At the same time, I felt like I had a major responsibility in taking care of my patients. I had a major responsibility in trying to recruit other young African-American physicians as well. There are not many of us. In medical school there were three black males in my class of more than 130 students. In my residency there is a decent number, but there still are not many of us. I mentor pre-med students, I have some of them shadow me in the emergency departments, I talk to junior residents. I have recruited for my residency program because these same things were done to me, and that is one of the reasons that I am actually doing emergency medicine. The orthopedic surgeon I saw when I was 16 or 17 years old was also African-American, and he took an active interest in me to make sure that I got to this point.

Having mentors and talking to people who are going to be supportive is extremely important. You do not want someone who is going to lie to you or feed you false information, but I think it is important that you have someone who is going to be encouraging and supportive of your dream.

How have you grown professionally and personally during your residency?

I think I have gotten more organized. I have become more responsible. This is stuff that is developed even more over the chief year. You have all the responsibilities: you are helping make sure that other residents in your program have certain things that are carried out, from the scheduling, making sure that certain lectures that you provide for the residents are up to par so they benefit from that. You have so much on your plate that you do not have a choice but to become better organized.

I have learned to take it easy, and to step back from situations when things are getting very hectic. Medicine is a challenging profession and it can consume you. A lot of physicians — a lot of people in general in many professions — do not have an outlet, and I think it is important for you to have some sort of outlet, or an escape from your regular, day-to-day duties, so that you can get out of that situation, and you can reflect upon it, and when you do get back to work, you feel somewhat refreshed, or at least have a clear mind.

I have been studying martial arts for a few years. I also run, and it helps me clear my mind. When I do not do those things, I can get irritable [laughs], I can get angry, and I realize that and think, "What is going on?" And I realize, you know what, I have not worked out in a couple days. When I train in my class, I am not around other physicians, so we do not talk about medicine. When I go out for my run, I do not have to have conversations with anybody else. I can meditate and reflect on things that have happened to me throughout the day or throughout the week.

What is it like being a chief resident?

We have about 54 residents in our program and two senior residents are chosen as chief residents. You let your program director know that you are interested in becoming a chief resident, and you are selected by the faculty as well as the senior residency class. As chief resident, there are a number of different duties. We do the scheduling for when the residents are in the ER. We do a lot of teaching. We do a lot of administrative work, behind-the-scenes stuff that I just never really realized [laughs] chief residents did. We sit in on faculty meetings; we are involved in the emergency services meetings as well. We do a lot of recruitment. During interview season, we set up a lot of stuff for the interview candidates.

Our days can vary. We have a specific number of emergency medicine shifts that you have to do per month when you are in the ER, and our shifts are eight to nine hours. So once your shift is done, you go home. It can be a day shift from 8:00 a.m. to 4:00 p.m., it can be an evening shift, 4:00 p.m. to midnight, or a night shift, midnight to 8:00 a.m. When you are done, you go home unless you have a lecture, and then you go to the lecture for a couple hours. After that you may go to work if you are scheduled to work for that day, or you go home and crash for the next seven to eight hours, if you have worked overnight. When I have a non-clinical day, you know, as a chief resident, I have a number of office duties. Sometimes I do that at the office, sometimes I stay home and work from my computer.

What is it like working in an emergency room?

We try to call that organized confusion [laughs]. It is organized in terms of the structure, but sometimes it can be called confusing or chaotic because you never really know what to expect. Some days may be very low-key or very low-stress: your patients are behaving very appropriately, no one is talking out loud to himself/herself or talking to the wall [laughs]. Some of the problems may not be that complex, but then, in a matter of five to 10 minutes, things can completely change.

We take care of almost any given emergency, from chest pains to patients having difficulty breathing. We take care of patients who have lacerations or major cuts to their extremities or to their bodies. We take care of patients who may have gynecologic problems: patients in their first trimester of pregnancy that may be having complications from that. We take care of patients who may be septic and they have bacteria in their blood; we take care of patients who come from all over the world; we take care of cancer patients; we take care of patients with almost every disease known to man. In our emergency department, I have seen leprosy.

In Cook County Hospital, one of the perks of working there is that it is a major emergency department and we do have a very large international population that comes through our emergency department so you see diseases from all over the world. It is kind of nice when you sit down to do your regular reading from your textbook and you go, "Wow, you know what? I saw this last week." That happens more often than not. We also take care of trauma patients as well — people who have been in car accidents, people who have been shot, people who have been stabbed.

Who has been influential to you during your residency?

I would have to say my program director, Dr. Steve Bowman. He is also my official faculty mentor, which helps. He has just been very helpful throughout my residency, from giving advice on lectures to giving personal advice.

What advice would you give to medical school graduates who are starting their residencies?

I would say take some time out for yourself, initially. Residency is a long time. The last thing you want to do is start that period of your life stressed out. Take a trip. Spend some time with your family. Go to the mountains, go to another country. It is not the last time you can take a trip like that, but I think it is something that will provide a certain amount of tranquility before you start a very hectic schedule.

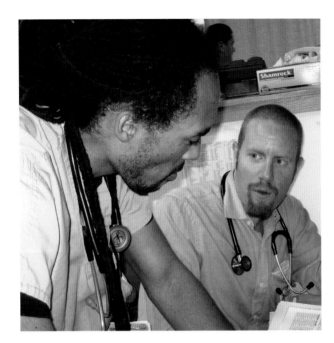
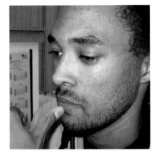
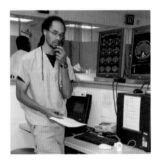

"MEDICINE SHOULD NOT JUST BE YOUR PROFESSION OR YOUR JOB – IT SHOULD BE YOUR CALLING."

Take your time and really talk to people about the specialty that you decide to choose. Many people decide on specialties because they watch television programs and they say, "Oh, okay, that is what I am supposed to do." Get involved, join organizations and interest groups for specific specialties and get exposure to those specialties early on. That way, when you do start that program, it is not a complete shock to your system. Unfortunately, there are a lot of residents who start residency programs and realize, "You know what? This is not for me."

Some people choose specialties because they know they can make a lot of money. Other people choose specialties because someone kind of pushed them to do that. Mom or dad may have been a particular practitioner and they decide to follow in mom or dad's footsteps because it is expected of them. And that is fine, but you do not want to be unhappy with your specialty. It should be something you enjoy doing; it should be something that you see yourself doing for a long period of time

What is one thing that you think needs to be changed or improved in medicine? What is one thing that you think medicine does especially well?

One thing that I thought needed to be changed in medicine would be our work-hour issue, and that is something that has improved a lot. I think it was my second year of residency when the ACGME passed guidelines stating that residents could not go over 80 hours a week.

That was nationwide. I think that helped a *whole* lot. During residency, you are tired. And when you are even more tired, you make a lot of mistakes. We are fortunate to be taking care of patients, and the last thing that you want to do is make a really bad mistake on a patient that you are taking care of, because you were half asleep and you could not remember the dosages of a specific medication or you could not remember how to do something. We cannot just erase something and say, "Oh, sorry, I just made a mistake." People's lives are at stake, so taking your time and being coherent when you do specific things is extremely important.

In emergency medicine, we are really good about not going over the work hours that we are supposed to have for a given week. After eight or nine hours, you are tired, but you can go home, you can relax, and then you can recuperate and do something else. I think medicine does well making sure that physicians are able to communicate well with their patients. In the past, physicians in training may not have seen a patient until their third year in medical school. Now first-year medical students learn how to interview patients and I think it benefits the patient in the long run, because by the time you become a physician, you are comfortable talking to patients, and it is not something you are struggling with.

What are your career plans after graduation?

I am going to be an attending at Kings County Hospital in Brooklyn. I grew up in the area. It is a *huge* level one trauma center. It has a huge international population. It is almost a parallel universe to Cook County. It is also an academic institution, so I want to teach.

Is there anything else you want to say about your residency?

I would just say to other future residents to make sure you are happy with your decision. Medicine is going to be a big part of your life; you might as well be happy with it. It should not just be your profession or your job — it should be your calling.

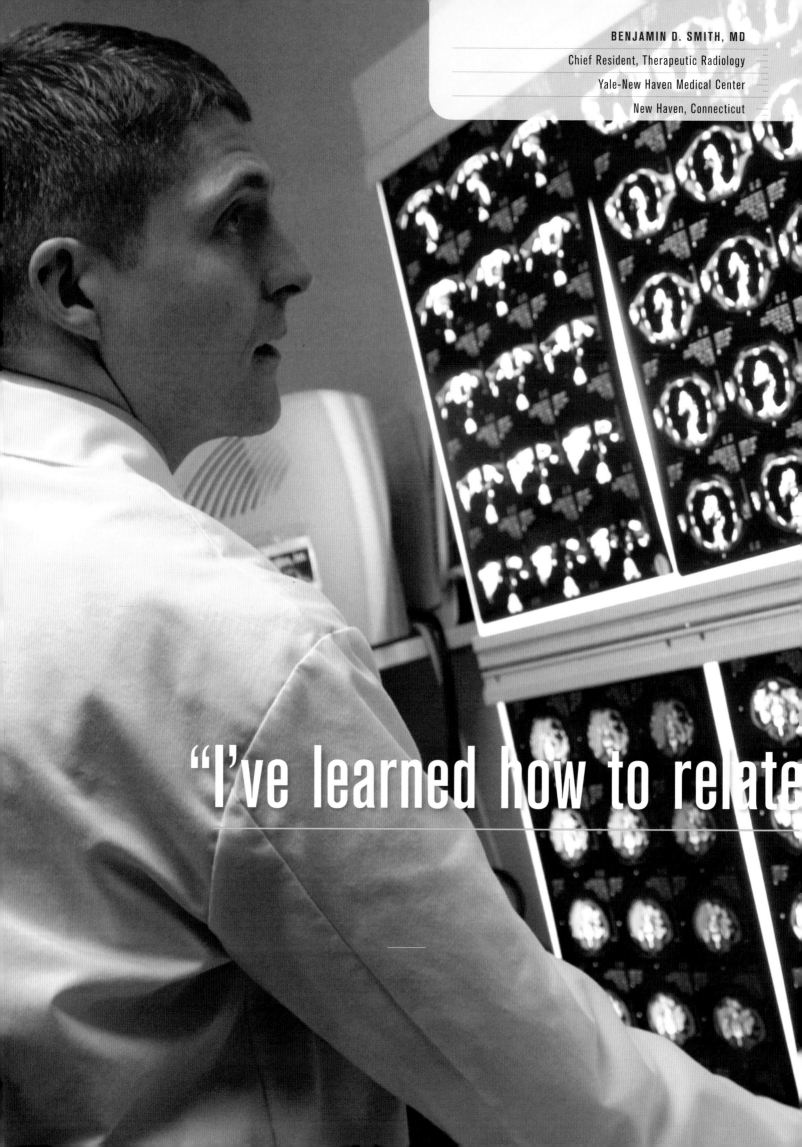

BENJAMIN D. SMITH, MD

Chief Resident, Therapeutic Radiology

Yale-New Haven Medical Center

New Haven, Connecticut

"I've learned how to relate

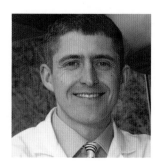

B enjamin Smith, MD, served as chief resident in radiation oncology at Yale-New Haven Medical Center in 2005–06, where the specialty is known as therapeutic radiology. Dr. Smith grew up in southern California, Oregon and Illinois, but decided to attend Rice University in Houston because of its strong program in engineering. However, he quickly discovered that medicine was his true calling.

In medical school, also at Yale, Dr. Smith was awarded the American Cancer Society Prize for his thesis on molecular markers in the treatment of head and neck cancers, as well as an award given to a graduating medical student who best exemplifies the Hippocratic Oath.

Dr. Smith, a captain in the Air Force Reserves, will serve for four years as a radiation oncologist at Wilford Hall Medical Center at Lackland Air Force Base in San Antonio, Texas, before entering an academic practice. Dr. Smith, who is married, also enjoys singing and jogging.

What attracted you to medicine?

I had always been interested in science, both physical sciences and biological sciences. When I went to college, I picked a college with a good engineering school because I intended to become a biomedical engineer. I had an internship in biomedical engineering the summer after my freshman year, and I found that although it was fascinating, I didn't find interacting with only a computer 40 hours a week to be personally gratifying. At that point I started thinking of a career in medicine that would allow me to bridge my passion for science with my passion to work with people and specifically to partner with them in times of suffering and need.

to people who have cancer."

I came to Yale medical school, graduated in 2001, and decided to stay at Yale for residency. I was very impressed by the quality of leadership at Yale, particularly the dean of students, and the strong commitment to education. Also, Yale has a very unique educational philosophy. At the medical school here there are no official grades for the first two years and the tests are anonymous. For me that was the perfect educational environment because it gave me the freedom to invest in things I was really passionate about and, as a result, as a medical student I was able to do a great deal of cancer research and publish several research articles and review articles.

Photographs: Terry Dagradi, MedMedia Group, Yale School of Medicine

When did you decide you wanted to go into radiation oncology?

Initially I had a strong interest in cancer and wanted to be a surgical oncologist, perhaps a head and neck surgeon dealing with head and neck cancers. Initially, I had planned to apply in otolaryngology programs. In my fourth year of medical school, I found that otolaryngology would not be an option for me due to my service obligation to the U.S. Air Force. So, literally, at the last minute in my fourth year of medical school I had to pick another specialty, and radiation oncology was a natural choice for me because I had done research with the program director right here in the department of radiation oncology.

What was the first day of your residency like?

I was scared to death. I started my internship in the intensive care unit [a one-year residency is required in internal medicine before beginning a radiation oncology residency], and I was on call my first day. I regarded that as a baptism of fire. It was very terrifying to all of a sudden call myself a physician in front of patients and to assume physician-like responsibilities for my patients. Thankfully, most of the physicians that I worked with at Yale were extremely supportive and really helped to smooth that transition. After a few weeks, being an intern was no longer terrifying; I started to gain competence in performing my basic duties.

However, internship remained very challenging, as the internship program here at Yale was extremely intense. I had to work the first 36 days without a day off, and I was on call every third or fourth night. Physically, I found it extremely exhausting. That was before any regulations regarding duty hours [the ACGME common duty hour standards that took effect in July 2003]. Things have changed a lot here at Yale since then.

Is there anything from your internship year that stands out in your memory?

For me the most positive aspect of internship was the opportunity to work with some extremely stellar co-interns, residents, chief residents and attendings. I was very happy to feel that I worked with a set of colleagues in whom I had complete trust regarding their ability to care for patients and from whom I learned a tremendous amount about being a doctor, both in interpersonal aspects of being a physician and day-to-day clinical decision-making.

It was really exciting to view my four years of college, four years of medical school, and one year of internship culminating in beginning a residency program in radiation oncology. I was very excited to learn this field, and I was very fortunate that I stayed to do residency in the same medical school where I had been a medical student and intern. In some ways I felt like I was coming home because I was working with the same people I had worked with throughout medical school.

Describe some of the things you do in your residency.

We see patients in clinic, and we do complete histories and physicals on them. We talk to them about the type of cancer they have and whether or not we think they would benefit from radiation therapy. We have long discussions with our patients regarding what is going on with their health in general and their cancer and how radiation fits in with the overall treatment program for their cancer. If we think the patient would benefit from radiation, we discuss the risks and benefits of radiation, and, if they agree to proceed, there is a large technical component to planning radiation therapy.

We map out the radiation treatment in a process called simulation, which typically involves a CAT scan, and there's a fair amount of behind the scenes work where we select the right size of the beams and the angles of the beam. We work with specialists in radiation physics to optimize the radiation treatment plan. During that course of radiation therapy, which can last anywhere from four to eight weeks, we provide our patients with medical care to address side effects that may arise. In general, people develop fatigue from the treatment. People can develop a skin reaction; for example, when we treat patients with breast cancer, they may develop a mild to severe skin reaction. Sometimes that skin reaction places them at risk for infection. Patients can develop a whole host of problems related to cancer: blood clots, low sodium, high calcium levels, and a number of different problems that we help to evaluate and then help to get the patient triaged if he/she needs hospitalization, emergency care, or simply support in our ambulatory clinic. Also, many patients have cancer-related pain, so we do a lot of pain management.

What moments in your chief residency year have been particularly meaningful?

We have a number of students who are applying for residencies. It's been gratifying to develop relationships with these medical students. Two have worked with me on research projects, and several of the medical students have come to me for advice as they think about where to apply for radiation oncology residency programs. A couple of them have mentioned me in their interviews as a mentor who has helped them on their journey to become radiation oncologists, and that has been particularly gratifying. Part of the blessing and part of the power [of mentoring] is the ability to shape the next generation of physicians, people who will not just advance the field, but who may provide care to me, my family and friends in the future.

We recently saw a patient with metastatic prostate cancer, who had tremendous pain from a mass growing in his pelvic region. My attending was not sure if we could deliver a meaningful dose of radiation safely to alleviate his pain, given the prior radiation treatment this patient had received. I thought that perhaps using very sophisticated new radiation therapies, we could, and the attending challenged me to do it in coordination with the radiation physics team. We spent a fair amount of time working on a plan for this patient in order to deliver a meaningful yet safe radiation dose. The patient ultimately passed away from his cancer, yet his pain had resolved prior to his death. It was gratifying to use new technology in a way that provided a meaningful benefit for this patient.

What do you do as a chief resident?

In our program, the historical standard is that all residents in their senior year share the responsibility of being the chief resident. In my year, there are two other residents, and we share the job of chief resident. We work really well together; they are fantastic people.

Part of it is administrative duties — the rotation schedule, the call schedule, the vacation schedule, those sorts of issues that are relatively mundane.

All three of us who are chief residents have taken a very strong interest in improving the resident teaching in our department. Every week we have a disease site that we plan to discuss. We select key articles about the specific cancer that we would like to discuss, and we e-mail those to the other residents and we go over them together, and we highlight key clinical concepts for the more junior-level residents.

How have you grown professionally and personally?

Professionally, it is easy to answer that question. When I first began residency in radiation oncology, I would listen to the senior residents discuss clinical issues, and I would think to myself "Will I ever know as much as this person about radiation oncology?" and now that I am at the end of my residency, I feel like I really have a good handle on the basic clinical applications of radiation therapy. I feel confident to begin my practice as an independent radiation oncology attending, so that is extremely exciting for me.

Personally, I have also grown. I've learned, sometimes through my own mistakes, how to relate to people who have cancer in a way that can be both truthful about the underlying disease process, yet also offer a sense of hope and encouragement to them. I have also learned to be more comfortable saying when I don't know the answer to patients and other physicians and to feel comfortable knowing my own limitations and knowing when I need to ask other people for help or to look things up before making a judgment or statement.

Emotionally, it is very draining, if you truly want to walk with your patients and show compassion for them. It is discouraging when they don't do well, and it is truly sad. It is very important to structure your life so there is a balance of both giving to patients and also taking time for yourself that renews your own soul.

What do you want to do after your Air Force service?

My career goal is to become a professor of radiation oncology at a high-quality academic medical center. My goals are to develop a strong mentorship relationship with residents and medical students, and ideally I would be very interested in becoming a program director of a radiation oncology residency program in the future. I would also like to build a clinical research career. I have some interest in both breast cancer and lymphoma and would be interested developing clinical expertise in one of these.

Who was most influential to you during your residency?

There have been a number of people who have been influential. I became a radiation oncologist because of the positive interactions I had with our former program director, Dr. Bruce Haffty. He was my thesis advisor during medical school, and he was the initial person who encouraged me to consider radiation oncology. I owe my residency position to him, thanks to the recommendation he submitted five years ago.

My wife has been an amazing mentor to me throughout my medical career. She is also a physician and is an intern in the department of internal medicine here at Yale. She is also working on completing her PhD in epidemiology. She has taught me how to do clinical research and has given me unbelievable advice in learning the details of statistical programming and statistical data analysis and learning how to craft a paper so that it will be reviewed favorably. She is a wonderful sounding board with whom I discuss clinical issues, and she provides me with encouragement and wonderful advice as I try to become a better doctor.

What advice would you give to medical school graduates who are starting their residencies?

It is critically important to identify a field in medicine in which you have a driving passion, and once you have identified that field, to think about how you can leave that field stronger than it was when you first began in the field. For example, if you have a passion for teaching, how can you make your teaching program stronger? If you excel at basic science research, how can you join a team of cutting-edge researchers and address cutting-edge questions? Or, if you have passion for clinical research, how can you define important unanswered questions in your field and use creative thinking to address those questions?

What does medicine do particularly well and what can be improved?

In my generation, we are seeing tremendous advances in our understanding of medicine from a molecular standpoint, specifically in oncology. Really, a revolution is taking place before our eyes as we see the first targeted therapies make their way from the bench to the bedside.

As ways that medicine perhaps still has some room to grow, I was thinking that I would like to see greater integration of the physical care we provide with spiritual and emotional care. So many of the issues we confront as physicians have powerful spiritual dimensions; for example, patients who are non-compliant with their medical regimens perhaps due to social issues or perhaps personality disorders or families who are struggling with loss, grief and death. I'm not sure if we as physicians do a very good job in addressing these issues in our therapeutic plans for patients and fully incorporating other providers with expertise in those areas as we think about caring for the whole person.

Any other thoughts about your residency?

This process of starting as a first-year medical student and now being on the cusp of finishing my training is a tremendously gratifying experience. When I began at Yale, I knew so little about how the human body works, disease, and how to care for people who are suffering and ill. Now, I am leaving shortly with a well-developed tool chest of skills to help alleviate suffering in this world and to help cure people who have cancer. It is just a tremendously gratifying feeling. I feel the last nine years of my life have been well spent, and I look forward to having the blessing of practicing medicine, hopefully for many years to come.

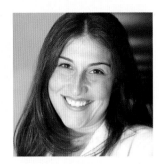

The father of Jill Weinstein, MD, is a physician, so medicine has always been part of her life. Still, although she liked science, she did not settle on a career in medicine until she was in college. Because Dr. Weinstein also has a passion for art, the mixture of science and artistry that is needed in dermatology drew her to the field.

After completing her residency, the Chicago native moved to Seattle with her fiancé, also a physician, and joined a multispecialty physicians' practice.

Why did you decide to become a physician?

I was not someone who knew at an early age that I wanted to go into medicine, but I really always liked science and the scientific method of thinking. My father was a physician specializing in infectious diseases, and growing up, I went to work with him and did experiments for science projects in his lab. He has been a great mentor and teacher throughout my medical career and someone I always look to for advice and guidance.

"You need to be able

I majored in biology as an undergraduate at Duke University. I spent time doing research projects and volunteering in the hospital in the early part of college and decided at that time that a career in medicine best suited my interests.

In addition to my interest in science, I have always had an interest in art. I took extra art classes in high school and college and enjoy the visual analysis as well as the creative aspects of art.

The summer before medical school I did research at the Northwestern Institute of Research and Policy Studies, and the physician in the office next door was a dermatologist who was studying skin cancer awareness and prevention. She told me that she loved her field because dermatologists have the ability to make such an impact on people's lives with small, relatively noninvasive procedures and that notion stuck with me. I got involved in a research project with her during my first year of medical school, and I realized that dermatology was a great fit for me. I particularly liked the fact that dermatology is a very visual field in which you see all ranges of patients and diseases but with a strong focus on preventive medicine.

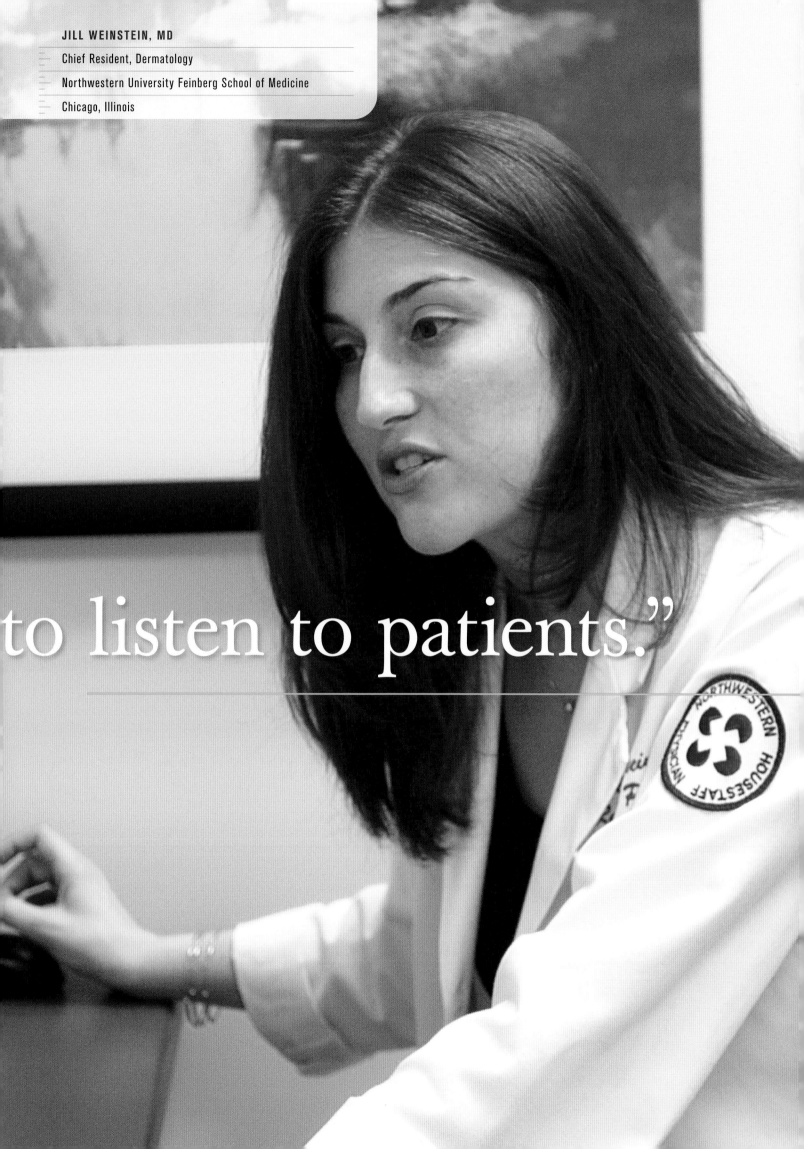

JILL WEINSTEIN, MD

Chief Resident, Dermatology

Northwestern University Feinberg School of Medicine

Chicago, Illinois

to listen to patients."

What stands out from the first year of your residency?

I did an internship in internal medicine in 2002 and started my dermatology residency in 2003. My internship was completely different from my dermatology residency yet they were both challenging in different ways. Internship was certainly daunting at first. As a medical student, someone is always watching over everything you do and you are protected in a way. As an intern, you have a lot more responsibility and a higher patient load. There is a steep learning curve.

The steep learning curve continued with my first year in dermatology. Dermatology is not taught a lot in medical school and comprises a week or less of the entire medical school curriculum. Consequently, I had a lot to learn, including basically an entirely new vocabulary used to accurately describe the things we see as dermatologists.

In my first year of dermatology residency, I did one of our most difficult rotations in the department of pediatric dermatology. I was responsible for seeing patients in clinic and in the hospital as well as phone triage and returning parent phone calls. Patients I saw had everything from congenital skin problems to severe eczema to vascular birthmarks to acne. A few weeks into the rotation, I remember getting a note from one of my attendings saying that I had responded to a difficult situation exactly how he would have responded. That gave me a sense of accomplishment, and I still have the note.

Did you feel confident that you would learn all you needed to learn to become a physician?

There is a lot to learn in dermatology and in medicine in general, but I have learned a great deal during my residency and feel confident in my ability as a dermatologist. Doctors are constantly learning new things, whether they are new interns, residents or the most senior attendings. I know I will continue to learn every day.

What is it like being a chief resident?

It is an appointed position, one resident out of the senior class. The attendings and other residents vote for the appointment. I was approached by the chairman to apply, but it was nothing that I had lobbied or asked for.

As the chief resident, I make up all the clinical schedules as well as the academic schedules, and I am the point person between all of the residents and all of the attendings. It has definitely been a challenge in my last year of residency to balance my administrative responsibilities with my need to solidify my knowledge base and develop my own personal style of practice. Having more responsibility forces you to be more efficient with your time.

How have you grown professionally and personally?

Professionally, I have acquired a tremendous fund of knowledge. Personally and professionally, I have learned how to interact with both colleagues and patients. In medical school you learn how to assess problems and make a diagnosis and learn a little bit about interacting with patients. A lot of your residency, in addition to learning more about medicine and your chosen specialty, is about learning how to interact with patients in a positive way, and I think that is one of the most important parts of a residency. You need to be able to listen to patients, not only to make a diagnosis and treatment plan, but to make sure they understand your thinking and make sure they do not leave the office wondering what is going on. Additionally, collaboration and constructive interaction with colleagues is very important during residency and beyond. The competitive atmosphere of medical school disappears, and everyone works together to make sure even the most complex patients are diagnosed and treated to the best of our abilities.

Who was the most influential to you during your residency?

In dermatology, we work with so many attendings who have different styles, different interests, and attract different types of patients that it really is hard to pinpoint one person. We have such an excellent clinical faculty and volunteer faculty at Northwestern. I really think I have learned from everyone I have worked with

What does medicine do well, and what can be improved?

One of the things that people in medicine do very well is continue to question. We are constantly trying to make sure that the knowledge we have is well supported and trying to find the answers to all the new questions that arise as a result of that knowledge. The research and technological advances that I have seen in my short career since I started medical school eight years ago have been astounding.

However, all of the research we do and new technology we create is not without a very high price. In an ideal world you want to expand coverage for everyone without compromising care or increasing costs, so that every patient would be able to benefit from everything we know about diagnosis and treatment of medical problems. Thus far, however, no one has been able to find a way for that to happen. Another thing that is unfortunate about the way we practice medicine is that liability issues have so much impact on how we practice. While it is important to have a system of checks and balances, I think a lot of what we do is out of fear of being sued, which is not the ideal approach to medicine.

What advice would you give to physicians starting their residencies?

Going from being a medical student to being an intern or resident can be a very tough transition, but in the end, it is a great feeling of accomplishment to be able to use everything that you have learned to care for your patients. It is important to learn to be responsible for your actions and decisions, and at the same time to know that you can always — and should often — ask for help or advice from your colleagues. Finally, despite the fact that there are not as many formal exams after medical school, it is important to remember that the best physician is one who continues to learn and stay current with the newest advances in medicine.

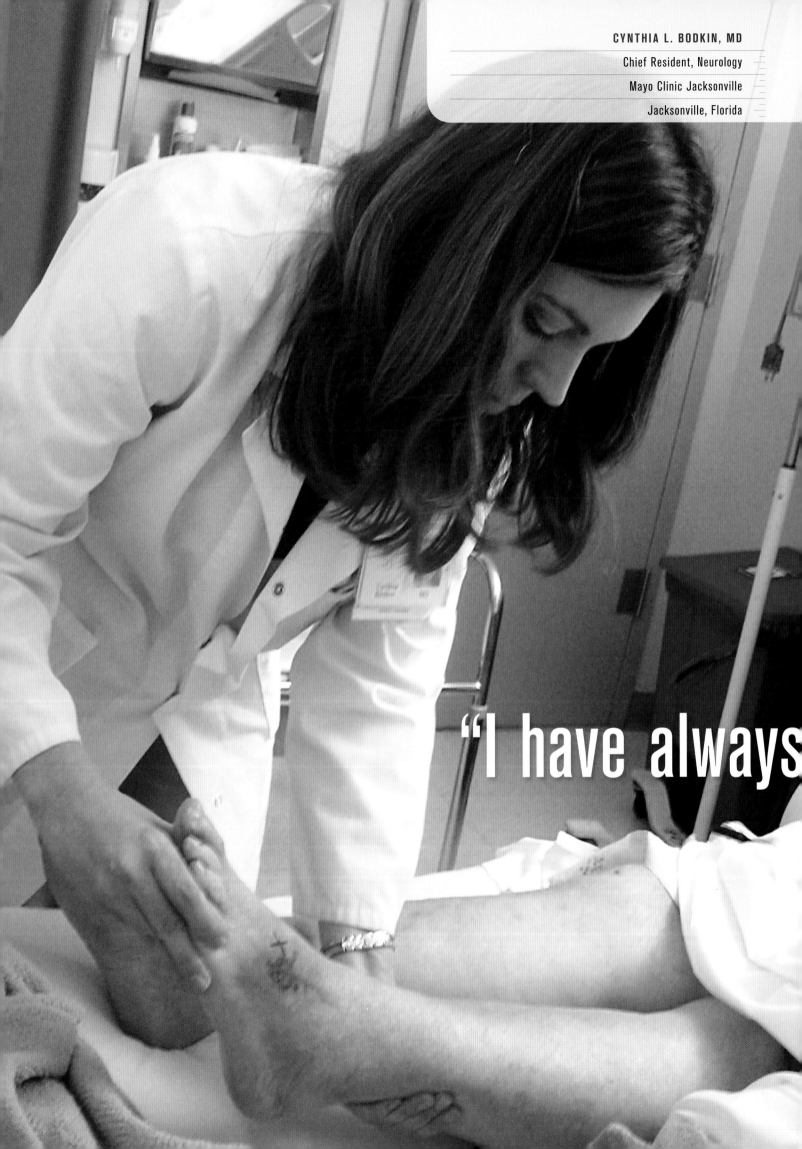

CYNTHIA L. BODKIN, MD

Chief Resident, Neurology

Mayo Clinic Jacksonville

Jacksonville, Florida

"I have always

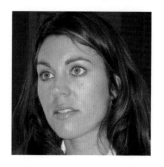

I t was the combination of analytical thinking and personal contact that attracted Cynthia Bodkin, MD, to neurology. Dr. Bodkin was one of two chief residents in neurology at Mayo Clinic Jacksonville during 2005–06. Dr. Bodkin, a native of Rochester, New York, earned a bachelor's degree in biology from Cornell University, and then went on to medical school at the State University of New York at Upstate Medical Center in Syracuse, New York.

Dr. Bodkin enjoys traveling, movies, rollerblading and spending time with family and friends. She is a member of the ACGME's Council of Review Committee Residents and a resident member of the Residency Review Committee for Neurology.

Why did you decide to become a physician?

Growing up I really never thought of a career in medicine. I did however want to do medical research in neurology. As an undergraduate, I quickly learned that basic science research was not the career choice for me. I didn't like the idea of being in a lab all day and never really interacting with a number of people. I felt locked away. So when I realized that basic science research was not for me in my sophomore year in college, I had to reexamine what career path I would take. I still enjoyed biology and other sciences, but wanted a career that included working with people. During this period in my life, someone mentioned medicine. It's like a light bulb went on. Medicine allowed me to put my desire to help and serve others with my love for biology. This was a perfect match for me.

found neurology fascinating."

What attracted you to neurology?

I always have found neurology fascinating. As I already mentioned, when I was younger I wanted to do research in neurology. Through the years I had wandered off the path of neurology. Going into medical school, I originally thought I would go into pathology. Then I took histology and the microscope gave me headaches and made me nauseated. There was no way I could spend a career looking in the microscope. At the same time I was taking histology I took neuroscience. I really enjoyed the logic behind neurology. Because I enjoyed neuroscience so much, I made sure I took my neurology clerkship early on in my third year of medical school. Once I completed my clerkship I knew I wanted to go into neurology. It was a rotation that I could not learn enough. Neurology is a field that depends heavily on the interactions of the physician and patient. From just the history and physical, I should be able to localize the medical problem. The thought process that goes into caring for a neurology patient is the type of medicine that I enjoy.

Mayo Clinic Jacksonville was my top choice for neurology. When I interviewed here the staff sold the program to us. They were clearly dedicated to the program and to making the residents great clinicians. At other programs I interviewed, you were in a herd of people; you never got to talk to any one person for a significant length of time. Mayo Clinic was much different. I felt that they truly wanted to know me and not just my scores.

What did you feel like on your first day of your transitional year residency?

Definitely extremely nervous. Very anxious. Excited in some way, but at the same time scared to death that I was going to make a mistake, that I was going to cause harm to somebody, or that people were going to know that I didn't know what I was doing. However, it didn't take long to realize that there was a lot of supervision, a lot of people making sure I did the right things and teaching me what to do. After the first week I realized it was not as scary as I thought and that I did actually know something about medicine.

Is there any moment that stands out from the first year of your neurology residency?

I can remember one night on call when it was very busy. The patients were admitted all at once, and we basically saw them and wrote orders. We finally sat down around 3 a.m. to write our notes on the patients that had been admitted early. I was an intern at that time, and one of the patients had a neurological complaint. However, the main reason the patient came in was for a GI bleed, which we were treating appropriately. I then started addressing other issues that weren't as critical but definitely part of his reason for coming to the hospital. And at that point my senior just looked at me and said, "I have no idea what to do. I'll just let you go with the plan you had already come up with." He just started laughing He was very honest. The patient had a weird movement disorder, and my senior let me order the tests I wanted, which isn't really much in the middle of the night. This was toward the end of the year, and I felt that I knew more about neurology than my senior medicine resident. It kind of felt good.

When did you start feeling like a real doctor?

I think the first time I really realized it was the following year when the new interns started out. You realize how little they know, and realize "I was just like that, and look how much I know now." That's when I really realized how much I was learning and how confidant I was about things they were still nervous about.

How is the chief year the same and different from the first year of your residency?

There are a lot of similarities. I still do similar call as I did as a PGY-2 [post-graduate year two] I am still seeing the same type of patients and caring for them, except I have more confidence and knowledge in what I am doing. At the same time, in the chief role, there are more administrative things as well, like the call schedule, arranging for journal club and lectures, and dealing with problems arising among residents, which luckily for us haven't been really any.

Do you mentor the other residents?

We definitely do play a role in teaching, getting articles, showing them how to do exams and procedures. I enjoy the teaching aspect of it. However, it is more stressful when you have to give some responsibility to the PGY-2. It took a while to get used to how to supervise them without their feeling like you don't trust them, but at the same time keeping an eye out so that they don't do anything that will harm a patient. It is nerve-wracking and a little more work in the beginning because you are always overlooking what they are doing. As the year goes on, you see them progress. Their knowledge expands and you begin to feel comfortable with their knowledge and judgment.

How have you grown both as a person and a physician?

Over the past four years, I have definitely become more confident in my knowledge and my skills. Even patients in my continuity clinic that I've followed for the past three years have said that I've become an excellent physician. My confidence, bedside manner, and, specifically, my ability to discuss the disease process and prognosis have all grown. This is very important in neurology because, unfortunately, there are a lot of aspects of neurology where we don't have a lot of good treatments and many of the diseases are pretty disabling and severe. It takes a lot to be able to sit down with a patient and family and break the horrible news in an empathetic, compassionate way. Although I've grown as a physician, I still dread having to give bad news to patients and family. But at the same time, I feel more confident in my ability to have the difficult discussions and answer their questions.

The growth I have made as a person is hard to put into words. I look at life differently now. Things that would have upset me or stressed me out in the past don't seem that important now. I also cherish my time with family and friends more. I did not realize the importance of the time spent with friends and family until I was too busy to see them. It is easy in medical school to put your life on hold for your studies. In residency it is even easier to put all your time and energy into caring for a patient. However, I learned that my family and friends are just as important as my patients. I cannot put my life on hold for too long. There will always be ill patients to take care of, and therefore I needed to learn how to balance my life now.

What conversations with patients or their families are particularly meaningful?

There are definitely times, especially in hospital neurology, where we have to have difficult conversations with the family of severely injured patients. It may be brain death, a vegetative state or severe brain injury. As a team we will sit down and talk with the family. We explain what happened and the prognosis. Not that it is rewarding when the family is crying, but when they thank you for being honest with them and telling them up front, although it is horrible what you're telling them, at least we are not making a horrible situation even worse for the family by not giving them all the information and not being honest with them.

What are your plans after graduation?

I will be doing a clinical neurophysiology fellowship here at Mayo Clinic Jacksonville. I am looking more toward the academic aspect of neurology. I really do enjoy teaching, and I also enjoy having colleagues who are experts in other fields.

Do you feel confident in your ability to practice independently?

I do understand in medicine that I will never be able to know everything, but I definitely feel I have the knowledge to treat the common things. I also know where my limitations are and where to look in order to get the information I need on the rare diseases. I have learned a logical, systematic approach to evaluating every patient. I am able to obtain the history, exam, develop a differential, order the appropriate test to support the diagnosis and treat the illness when treatments are available. I have also developed experience in when things are an emergency and when I have time to ponder the patient's illness.

Who was a mentor to you during your residency?

It definitely would have to be Dr. Frank Rubino. He was one of the traditional, classic clinicians. His bedside manner can't be compared to anyone else's. When you look at a Norman Rockwell painting, Dr. Rubino would be the physician you would imagine. His clinical skills are excellent. He doesn't use the technology we have today to make diagnoses. He does it with the history and the exam, and then uses the technology, whether an MRI and CT scan, to confirm what he already knows. We tend to get into the habit now of ordering all the tests, and letting the tests tell us what the disease is, instead of letting us figure out the disease and using the tests to confirm what we know. Dr. Rubino was in charge of our continuity clinic. Some of the patients in the clinic had been his patients for years. The bond he had with his patients was amazing. His patients would travel here from other states just because of him and the bond they shared. His excellence doesn't stop at his clinical skills and his bedside manner. He was an excellent teacher. He would always say that there was no one he could not teach. Clearly in medicine not every physician has mastered the art of teaching, but Dr. Rubino did. I am lucky to have been one of the many residents Dr. Rubino has trained. I hope I can be half the clinician Dr. Rubino was and carry on his legacy.

Dr. David Capobianco [the program director] has also been very influential. He clearly supports the residents. The residents are his first priority. If there's any problem that needs to be addressed, we can count on him to be our advocate. He is also active nationally in neurology. He encourages us to take an active role as well. There are many opportunities for committees or awards where the program directors can nominate a resident. Unfortunately, a number of program directors never nominate anyone. Dr. Capobianco always take the opportunity to nominate a resident that he feels is worthy of the award, or if he knows a position is available on a committee, he lets the residents know about it.

What advice would you give to medical school graduates?

The main thing is not to be so nervous. They are going to be no matter what I say, but they should realize that most residency programs are out there to make sure you succeed as a

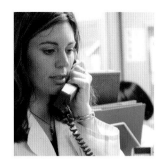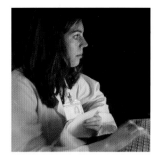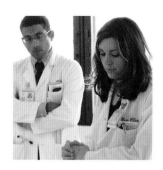

"I HAVE LEARNED A LOGICAL, SYSTEMATIC APPROACH TO EVALUATING EVERY PATIENT."

physician; they are not out to get you. The programs are going to be by your side to make sure you get the education you need. Also, you're not by yourself. There are physicians there you can look to for help.

I also would recommend, even though it is hard and very easy to lose track of time and to get swept up in medicine, that you also need to have a private life as well. You need to balance your life with your family and friends. Yes, there are always months where you get busy and lose track of time. However, over all the four years I have been here, I have had the time and ability to balance my life between my family and friends and my medical career.

What one thing in medicine would you like to change?

I don't know if it would be possible, but it would be great to order a test or treat a patient the way you feel is best for that patient without worrying if their insurance will cover the medications or tests, or what the patient can and can't afford. Unfortunately, with a lot of the seizure medications and other medications, there is variability in the cost and the coverage of health insurance for prescriptions. There are times where, although one medication may be better for the seizure disorder and not have as many side effects, if the patients can't afford it, they are not going take it, so you're better off to go with the cheaper medication that may have more side effects, but at least then you know they will be taking it.

I would also like to be able to order tests, or not order tests, just purely on my medical opinion. Unfortunately, the way malpractice has become, tests are done not because you feel the patient needs it but because of defensive medicine.

Is there anything else that you would like to say about being a chief resident?

It is an excellent experience. You definitely grow throughout the year. It is not as easy to supervise someone as you might think. There is a tight balance between supervision and micromanaging. It can be difficult to allow the junior resident to have some autonomy and growth at the same time you are growing as a chief. At the same time you gain a new type of respect for your attendings. As chief, you also begin to learn the complexity of the administrative work behind medicine. I feel I am a better physician from my experience as a chief.

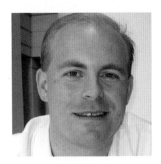

t was the analytical aspect of anesthesiology, as well as the opportunity to connect with patients, that appealed to Reed VanMatre, MD. Dr. VanMatre, a native of New Castle, Indiana, earned a degree in biomedical engineering from Northwestern University and then completed his medical degree at Northwestern University, Feinberg School of Medicine. He then entered the anesthesiology residency program at Duke University Medical Center in Durham, North Carolina.

In his free time, Dr. VanMatre enjoys woodworking and spending time outdoors with his wife, Gail, and their two dogs.

Why did you decide to go into medicine?

I decided to go into medicine when I was 17. I went through a combined bachelor's and MD program at Northwestern. I was interested in science. I was a person who enjoyed science classes at school and I wanted to go to college and study engineering. I worked as a pharmacy delivery boy in high school, and I really enjoyed meeting and talking with the elderly people on my route. That experience cemented my decision to work in a clinical setting, rather than an office or a laboratory. As a 17-year-old, the decision to go into medicine seemed perfectly natural. Now, at 30, I realize that I did not have much insight at that time into what it means to be a physician, but I am happier than ever with my decision. In retrospect, I would advise most high school students against making a commitment to a career path so early on.

"Plan ahead and pay

What attracted you to anesthesiology?

I really did not decide until the end of my third year in medical school, right before it was time to apply for residencies. I liked acute medicine. I thought of being an intensivist, and I really enjoyed the anesthesiologists whom I worked with in the ICU. I like thinking of and working with the body as a series of physiologic control systems. So that aspect of anesthesiology appealed to me. It is acute in nature and I have to interact with complex physiology on a regular basis. I like working with my hands in both my profession and hobbies — I like woodworking for example — and I wanted to do procedures on a daily basis. I am sort of a quiet person, and most of the anesthesiologists I met were quiet achievers. They were doing really great things but were not in the spotlight. That appealed to me — that I could be subtle but still do something really important and make a huge difference.

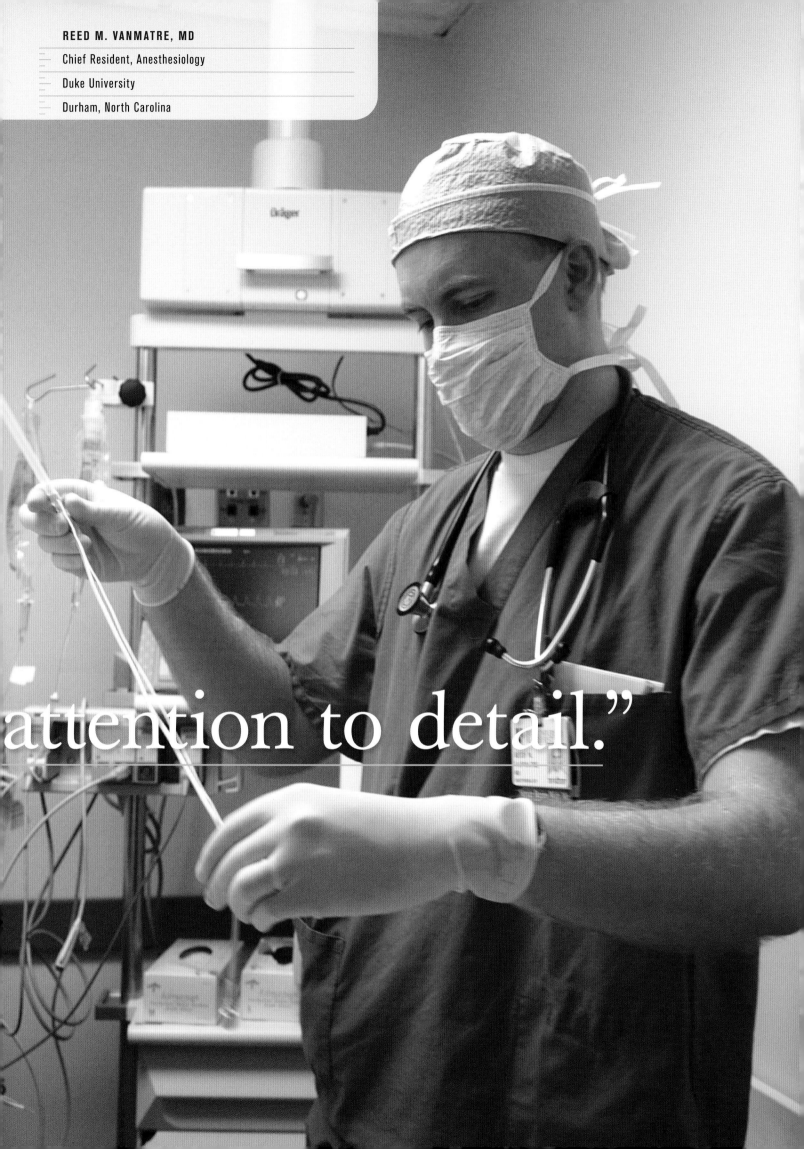

REED M. VANMATRE, MD

Chief Resident, Anesthesiology

Duke University

Durham, North Carolina

attention to detail."

Why did you choose Duke for your residency?

Before coming down here, I did not really know what to expect. What I found at Duke were people who were doing amazing things in terms of innovations in clinical care and research, but at the same time were very nice people. The environment was very warm and friendly. I liked the residents whom I met. I thought I would get great clinical experience here. If I wanted to get involved in research, there were numerous opportunities as well.

How did you feel on the first day of your residency?

I was not particularly scared, just a little intimidated. I was excited to be starting, and I was happy to be moving on to the next stage in my career. I felt like I was finally getting really close to doing what I had wanted to do for a long time.

Most of the anesthesiology residents here do a transitional year. It is an internship that combines months in different services — emergency medicine, intensive care, medicine, etc. An incident that sticks in my mind was the code pager going off during my first night on call in the surgical ICU. My most vivid recollection is the rush I felt running down the hall with the bright orange airway bag. I was finally doing what I had come to my residency to do, and what I wanted to do for the rest of my life — to help people who are acutely ill and in need of my urgent attention. That was amazing.

When did you first feel like a doctor?

I guess the first day of internship when I realized that even though there were people supervising me, I was the bottom line. Even though the nurses, respiratory therapists and others had worked at Duke for many years, they looked to me as the doctor. The feeling came more from others than it did from within.

Did you feel confident that you would learn all you needed to know?

Sure. At some point I realized that learning is a continuous process, and that this is just the beginning. We are all lifetime learners. That is comforting. Although, of course, I needed to know certain things to be a qualified, certified anesthesiologist, at some point, I realized I would continue to learn throughout my career, and I could not expect to learn everything within a discrete amount of time that was set aside for residency training. I had seen lots of people graduate and become competent physicians, and I did not feel the situation would be any different for me.

What is it like being a chief resident?

This is part of our last year of our residency. We do not spend an extra year as chief residents. It is mostly administrative. There are two chief residents each year — we each serve for six months. Most importantly, we are liaisons between the residents and department leadership. We meet regularly with the program director and department chairman and are integrated into the leadership circle. We disseminate information to the residents and solicit ideas from them that we can take back to the leaders. I was surprised at how much the leaders look to us for input. They expect us to have a finger on the pulse of the residency.

Anesthesiology is unique. We operate pretty independently as residents in comparison to, say, a medical team, where there is a senior resident, junior resident and intern. We end up working by ourselves under the supervision of an attending anesthesiologist. We do not have as much of an opportunity to mentor younger residents on a daily basis.

How have you grown as a person and a doctor?

I think all residents get a more realistic view of medicine during their training. We all start out being very idealistic. I do not think I have lost that much idealism, but I realize there are certain limits to what physicians can do, what we can and cannot achieve. At some point, we have to make tough decisions and admit that we cannot always win.

Have there been any moments this year that have been particularly meaningful to you as a chief resident?

Some of the most meaningful times were when I had the opportunity to help residents who were having problems with their personal lives or problems with the demands of the residency. If I could help them in the smallest way to feel valued or to help them deal with problems, that was really meaningful to me.

Who has been most influential person to you in your residency?

One of our pediatric anesthesiologists, Dr. Ryan Cook, who has been an anesthesiologist for nearly forty years, really took an interest in helping me grow as a physician. Once I became a chief resident, he helped me grow as a leader as well.

My program director, Dr. Catherine Lineberger, has also had a great deal of influence on me. She is an excellent clinician and teacher, a strong role model who is highly respected by her peers.

What are you going to do after your residency?

I have not really decided. I am doing a fellowship next year at Duke in cardiothoracic anesthesia. That will help me make my decision on where I want to go with my career.

What is one thing that medicine can improve, and one thing that medicine does very well?

Our health care system is a tremendous source of scientific development. One thing we do really well is to innovate and come up with exciting new therapies and ways to care for patients. On a more basic level, I think that preventive medicine and primary care are areas that deserve more attention and funding. Many of the patients whom I care for in the operating room would not be sick if they had received better preventive services earlier in life.

What advice would you give to physicians starting their residencies?

Life is a marathon, not a sprint. No matter how daunting the task, if you plan ahead, approach the problem systematically and pay attention to detail, you will be successful.

ABOUT THE PHOTOGRAPHER

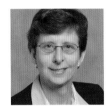

ROBERTA E. SONNINO, MD, is a pediatric surgeon and associate dean for academic and faculty affairs at Creighton University School of Medicine in Omaha, Nebraska. Dr. Sonnino has long been interested in photography and earned a certificate as a professional photographer from the New York Institute of Photography. She has her own freelance photography business, Hi RES Photos, www.hiresphotos.com. Her photography has been featured in the television show *Extreme Makeover Home Edition,* in a permanent exhibit at the Washington, DC headquarters of the AAMC, and on the cover of a recent book, *Ghost Plane,* published by St. Martin's Press. Dr. Sonnino has had three solo exhibits of her "Fragile Beginnings" series of medical photographs featuring many of her young patients.